W9-AHN-888

APPLYING QUALITY MANAGEMENT IN HEALTHCARE

A Process for Improvement

APPLYING QUALITY MANAGEMENT IN HEALTHCARE

A Process for Improvement

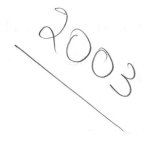

Diane L. Kelly

Health Administration Press, Chicago, Illinois
AUPHA Press, Washington, DC

AUPHA
HAP

Your board, staff, or clients may also benefit from this book's insight. For more information on quantity discounts, contact the Health Administration Press Marketing Manager at (312) 424-9470.

07   06   05   04   5   4   3   2

Library of Congress Cataloging-in-Publication Data
Kelly, Diane L.
    Applying quality management in healthcare : a process for improvement / Diane L. Kelly.
      p. cm.
    Includes bibliographical references and index.
    ISBN 1-56793-206-1 (alk. paper)
    1. Medical care—Quality control.   2. Health services administration.   3. Total quality management.   I. Title.

RA399 .A1K455 2003
362.1'0685—dc21   2003044998

Acquisitions editor: Audrey Kaufman; Project manager: Jane Williams

Health Administration Press
A division of the Foundation
  of the American College of
  Healthcare Executives
One North Franklin Street
Suite 1700
Chicago, IL 60606
(312) 424-2800

Association of University Programs
  in Health Administration
730 11th Street, NW
4th Floor
Washington, DC 20001
(202) 638-1448

To Dan and Anna

BRIEF CONTENTS

DETAILED CONTENTS

Section III Achieving Quality Results in Complex Systems

FOREWORD

In the Preface of *Striving Toward Improvement: Six Hospitals in Search of Quality* (JCAHO 1991), Don Berwick tells the story about mountaineering to demonstrate that managers need to learn the difference between method and result. Berwick says: "Obsession with results is the impediment to improvement . . . . How could a basketball team get better if the coach taught the players [to] . . . '[n]ever take your eyes off the score board'." Instead, Berwick points out: "[f]orget the scoreboard . . . study . . . the methods of play . . . how to hold the ball, where to place your hands . . . and how to learn how to learn on your own."

As the story goes, Berwick and a group of climbers met Phil Ershler, a world-class mountaineer who has stood on the summits of Mount Everest and K2. Ershler was to guide Berwick and the group on their climb to Mount Rainier, which is no Everest but is a serious mountain nonetheless. Although Berwick had climbed Mount Rainier several times before, he arrived at the top exhausted each time. Now Ershler was the guide on his fourth climb. Before the climb, Ershler said he was first going to teach Berwick and the group "how to walk and how to breathe." Berwick "thought he was crazy," and the group laughed, saying, "We are here to learn technique . . . not walking and breathing!" Six hours into the climb, Berwick and the group were no longer laughing, as "Phil had done exactly what he said."

Berwick reports that the habitual, unconscious actions of walking and breathing had been transformed into self-conscious, planned, placed, comprehended, and practiced tools for success on the mountain. The group learned the "rest step," the use of rhythms, the conservation of motion, the focus of attention, the alternatives in placement of the foot, and kicking and sliding at just the right time. The group studied equipment, the shape of snow, the position of hips and arms, and the optimal distances between members of the group. Walking and breathing, under Ershler's mentoring, had ceased being the simple, intuitive staggering and puffing of a neophyte with desperate eyes fixed on the summit. They had become a constellation of a dozen or more small and purposeful parts, each designed by experience, theory, and logic. Together, these learned parts added up to a new way, a transformation of methods. The next day of the climb, the group walked and breathed a new way. They arrived at their destination tested but fresh. Same mountain, new method, different experience.

This book is about how to walk and how to breathe. It focuses on the methods of quality management and their application within an organizational context. As with Berwick's mountain-climbing experience with Ershler, this book is not a comprehensive overview of various techniques but a systemic, integrated presentation of the fundamentals that managers need to know to make a difference in the practice of quality management. Each chapter is illustrated with relevant examples from the world of practice and is presented in an easy, readable manner. Exercises are included at the end of each chapter, providing the reader the opportunity to apply the concepts and methods discussed in the chapter. The chapters are presented in sequential form, building on fundamental concepts, underlying principles, and specific approaches for achieving quality results in complex systems.

However, the whole must be greater than the sum of its parts. Fulfilling this objective requires that the book provide an opportunity for the readers to synthesize the concepts, principles, and approaches. This opportunity can be found in the Epilog and in the Practice Exercises section in which three exercises are presented. The first one focuses on organizational assessment, the second on performance-improvement effort in a fictional organization with real-world conflicts, and the third on performance-improvement effort in an identified area in the reader's own organization.

Diane Kelly should be commended for a thoughtfully conceived and creatively crafted effort that will prepare managers with the skills necessary to improve the provision of health services. As well described by Edward Deming, a pioneer in quality improvement, "the problems are with the system, and the system belongs to management." In this book, Kelly has provided the opportunity for learning some methods that are analogous to Ershler's how-to-walk and how-to-breathe approach. These methods equip managers to address the problems and future challenges of the system for which they are the responsible agents.

Arnold D. Kaluzny, Ph.D.
Professor of Health Policy and Administration
School of Public Health
University of North Carolina at Chapel Hill

FOREWORD

The American healthcare system is currently facing increased scrutiny as a result of several high-profile reports that reveal that medical errors are common and have led to many patient deaths. In particular, the Institute of Medicine's (IOM) report, "To Err Is Human: Building a Safer Health System," has attracted much attention and commentary. IOM followed up this report with a series of publications that further focus on the safety and quality of care. Taken together, these reports have drawn considerable interest from all healthcare stakeholders, causing them to challenge the conventional wisdom that quality is a given in American healthcare today.

Quality of healthcare has been a recurring theme in the United States since the early part of the twentieth century, when the Flexner report, "Medical Education in the United States and Canada," which outlined the inadequacies of the medical education system, was published. This report ushered in an era of setting scientific standards and marked the beginning of the construction of the world's most sophisticated, technologically advanced, and expensive healthcare system. Given these beginnings and Americans' support of technological breakthroughs, it is understandable that a common assumption exists that the American healthcare system delivers the highest quality of care. This perception persists despite numerous scientific studies suggesting that the quality of care in the United States is highly variable and poorly measured.

As in other industries, public perception of the healthcare industry is often only altered by spectacular mishaps. Several recent notable accidents have contributed to an increased public awareness of the importance of quality in healthcare, such as the death of Betsy Lehman, the health editor of the *Boston Globe*, from an easily preventable overdose of a chemotherapy drug; the death of 8-year-old Ben Kolb from a drug mix-up during minor surgery; and the amputation of Willie King's good leg. Predictably, these and other such events have energized politicians, regulatory agencies, and industry and consumer groups to focus on improving quality in this area, with a resulting flurry of proclamations, legislative and regulatory activities, and reports on the subject. These activities in turn have energized the public to demand a much greater transparency for healthcare quality.

As such, JCAHO is now requiring healthcare delivery organizations to track and report inpatient processes and outcome measures that are indicative of quality; this information will soon be made public. In addition, other healthcare organizations—the American Hospital Association, the Centers for Medicare and Medicaid Services, and the Agency for Healthcare Research and Quality—have developed a voluntary quality-reporting initiative that allows hospitals to directly report certain quality measures for public availability; many similar efforts are ongoing. A tipping point has clearly been reached in providers' reporting of healthcare-quality information to the public. No longer will hospitals be able to use public-relations approaches to shape the public's view of the quality of care they provide. This information will now be controlled by other entities, creating a new era of accountability for the quality of care delivered by hospitals.

Although most healthcare delivery organizations can tell plenty of success stories surrounding their quality improvement efforts, many of these organizations have encountered barriers that have limited the impact of their quality efforts. These issues have included the cost of quality programs, the narrow impact of these programs, the inability to disseminate improvements throughout the organization, the difficulty of sustaining improvements, and the lack of true financial incentives in the marketplace for improved quality. Time and again, when these organizations get into financial difficulty, their quality programs are often the first to see reductions or elimination. Despite an increased focus on quality, many organizations are reeling from financial difficulties related to reimbursement issues, regulatory burdens, staffing shortages, and rising costs. It is fortuitous timing, as virtually all excess costs have been removed from most organizations through belt tightening; only a fundamental reappraisal of the processes of care, and of clinical processes in particular, can yield further significant savings while improving the quality of care. Nonetheless, without clear financial incentives, many organizations are hesitant to invest in new quality improvement programs.

Several new initiatives have begun addressing the issue of paying for better performance in safety and quality of care, the best example of which is the Leapfrog Group initiative. This group has developed three highly specific and well-publicized patient-safety standards that seek to financially reward publicly transparent hospital performance on these three standards. These standards have catalyzed significant interest and movement among hospitals in implementing these practices because of the impact on reimbursement. However, the Leapfrog Group's effort is not isolated; similar initiatives are also being implemented, such as the Pay for Performance Program in California and the Bridges to Excellence Program in the Midwest, which have begun to institutionalize the practice of better reimbursement for demonstrably higher quality care.

Timing is everything, and Diane Kelly's new book, *Applying Quality Management in Healthcare: A Process for Improvement,* arrives at a critical evolution point. As healthcare managers begin to see the impact of public demands for transparent accountability for quality, as regulators mandate the reporting of quality performance information, and as payers align reimbursement approaches to reward higher quality, they will need to quickly develop expertise in managing quality as a new skill set and ultimately as a core competency. To date, expertise and critical skills in this area have resided within the quality improvement or quality assurance department and occasionally within clinical departments. Managing the quality of care has not been a critical skill for healthcare management nor an inherent part of the manager's educational experience. However, these skills will quickly become an indispensable part of any manager's knowledge base. Rather than long-winded educational programs that revolve around theories of quality, managers will need a practical guide to quality that is long on examples, adequate on theory, and easy to understand from the management perspective—a how-to guide for managing quality. This is exactly what they will get from this book.

Not only does this book supply the fundamental theory that underlies successful management of quality, it also provides ample real-world examples and numerous exercises to help the reader quickly master the concepts. This book does not rehash old approaches in quality, but it picks up many of the fundamental issues and themes raised by IOM's reports. It offers an integrated approach to quality in complex systems that overcomes many of the inherent limitations of quality improvement in years past. Organizations would do well to use this book not only as a principal educational tool for managers but as a required one at that. Indeed, this book will quickly become the manager's healthcare quality survival guide.

In the past, organizations' focus was on marketing quality of care. In the future, it will be on delivering quality of care as part and parcel of the business operations of any successful healthcare delivery organization. Applying the principles and techniques in this new book is essential for any organization's continued existence.

David C. Classen, M.D., M.S.
Associate Professor of Medicine, University of Utah
Vice President, First Consulting Group
Salt Lake City, Utah

PREFACE

Applying Quality Management in Healthcare: A Process for Improvement is intended to help readers translate quality management theory and knowledge into practice. The book is easy to understand, and the real-life examples used to explain and illustrate technically complex concepts offer a highly leveraged approach to learning. Although the book does not provide comprehensive technical, medical, and policy background, it explores managerial and organizational issues related to healthcare quality to assist managers who are or will be operating in various levels and types of healthcare organizations.

Content Overview

The integrating theme of this book is systems thinking as it can be applied to healthcare organizations. Section I, "The Fundamentals of Quality Management," includes chapters that introduce concepts associated with quality management in healthcare and that explain common continuous quality improvement tools. Section II, "The Systems Approach," contains chapters that explore the influence of systems principles on quality management and that introduce the concepts of systems thinking and dynamic complexity as expressed in healthcare organizations. In this section, several system models are presented to help organizations understand how relationships among variables within the system influence their overall quality results. The final chapter in this section introduces the influences of systemic structure on sustainable improvement.

Chapters in Section III, "Achieving Quality Results in Complex Systems," explore assumptions around common management activities and functions. Alternative ways of thinking about topics such as goals, measurement, and implementation are presented to enhance the ability to achieve quality results. The Epilog synthesizes the information presented throughout the book. The Practice Exercise and Journal Exercise sections provide the opportunity to apply these concepts to real situations and settings.

The chapters are intended to be read in sequence, as current concepts are built on the previous concepts' foundation. However, individual chapters may be used to present stand-alone concepts. As the title implies, the selection of topics, the sequence of their presentation, and the types of learning exercises guide the reader through the process of learning and practicing quality management.

Levels of Learning

This book contains material developed for and taught at the University of North Carolina at Chapel Hill School of Public Health in the Department of Health Policy and Administration. The concepts and exercises have been tested in the classroom and refined over seven semesters of teaching master's-level students. These students include those from the residential master's program and the executive master's program; those with limited work experience and extensive work experience; those enrolled in a variety of programs, including the master of healthcare administration, the master of public health, and the master in nursing administration; and those with nonclinical backgrounds. Physicians, nurses, respiratory therapists, occupational therapists, and nutritionists were also part of the test groups.

Appropriate for healthcare administration students and practicing healthcare managers, this book offers readers different levels of learning according to the reader's needs, experiences, and circumstances. The first level of learning is attained by simply reading the chapter content; this will provide an overview of the concepts illustrated through real-life examples. The second level can be reached by reading the chapters and completing the end-of-chapter exercises; this level is appropriate for a practicing manager. The minimum level of learning recommended for healthcare administration students can be achieved by reading the chapters and companion readings and completing the end-of-chapter exercises. The recommended companion readings supplement the chapters by presenting more technical concepts. Instructors may choose to assign one, two, or all of the companion readings listed in each chapter.

The highest level of learning for both practicing managers and students is possible by adding a journal for each reading and completing the final exercises. The journal exercise is designed to allow readers (1) to reflect on the concepts presented in the chapter or reading, (2) to practice formulating effective management questions, and (3) to practice applying the concepts to real-world circumstances relevant to their own experience.

Acknowledgments

I extend my sincere gratitude to the individuals, teams, organizations, and students from whom and with whom I have learned over the years. Although it is impossible to list all of you by name, please know how important knowing and working with you has been to the collective lessons presented in this book.

A special thanks to several colleagues who have influenced my thinking about and practice of quality management and systems thinking: Thomas Petzinger, Jr., David Tew, Dorothy Weber, Stan Pestotnik, Michael Goodman, Brent James, David Classen, Donna Fosbinder, Marj Peck, and Jackie Mead. I also express my deepest gratitude to colleagues who have been a source of support, encouragement, and collaboration: Elizabeth Hammond, Lynnae Napoli, Marla Birch, Joan Lelis, Karie Minaga-Miya, Bill Shepley, Robert Crawford, Patty Silver, Robert Silver, Marlyn Conti, Nancy Short, Christie North, Joe Cramer, Melissa Zito, and Tim Empkie. I also acknowledge the important contribution of the University of North Carolina at Chapel Hill Public Health Leadership Program and its director, Bill Sollecito, to my academic and professional development.

I am indebted to my mentor, Dr. Arnold Kaluzny, whose support and belief in me made this book possible.

Diane L. Kelly, Dr.P.H, M.B.A, R.N.

THE FUNDAMENTALS OF QUALITY MANAGEMENT

CONCEPTS OF QUALITY MANAGEMENT

Objectives

*   To introduce the concept of quality from a healthcare manager's perspective
*   To define commonly used quality terms
*   To define quality management as used in this book
*   To describe a quality continuum for managers

A mother arrived at the pediatrician's office for her daughter's 6-month well-child check-up. As she had for previous check-ups, she arrived ten minutes early and requested to occupy the well-child waiting area so that her daughter would not pick up an infection from sick children in the regular waiting area. The scheduled appointment time of 10:00 a.m. passed, and so did 10:30, 11:00, and 11:30. The nurse politely told the mother that the pediatrician had been called to an emergency, saying, "I'm sure you understand. If it was your child, you would want the doctor to attend to her." Although the mother understood the reason for the delay, this explanation really did not help the fact that she had to pick up her son from preschool at noon. The mother hunted for the harried nurse, who was grabbing a bite of her lunch each time she passed the nurse's station, to ask if her daughter could receive the required immunization shots and to reschedule the rest of the check-up for another time.

Dissatisfied with the hours wasted at the pediatrician's office and disappointed with the need to return to finish the check-up, the mother asked if the pediatrician was on emergency call during the time of the rescheduled appointment. When the mother and daughter arrived for the follow-up appointment, the mother hovered over the receptionist's desk so that all of the staff knew that she was ready and waiting. The office staff quickly identified this mother as a "problem."

Because the child received her immunization shots and well-child care in accordance with the guidelines of the American Academy of Pediatrics, one may conclude that she and her family were given high-quality medical care. Although the medical interventions were thorough and carried out according to the best clinical evidence available, the lack of quality management is what caused this family's unsatisfactory interaction with the healthcare system. In this example, the lack of quality management is illustrated by the pediatrician being assigned to both well-child visits and emergencies on the same day, by ineffective patient scheduling and queuing systems, and by the poor mechanism with which the office communicates with patients and manages their expectations. These issues have nothing to do with the quality of the medical care; they have everything to do with the quality of the *patient's* care.

This example illustrates important questions healthcare managers today need to answer: What is quality? What is quality management? What is the manager's role in the quality process? This chapter will begin to address these questions by clarifying common concepts and defining terms typically associated with the word "quality" and how it is used and perceived in healthcare.

Management, as it occurs within the context of a healthcare organization, is the focus of this book. The material presented in this book is intended to provide managers with responses to the question, "What do I do now?" In other words, once policy decisions are made or clinical evidence is published, how do managers influence their own domain of organizational responsibility to ensure that policy requirements are met and that their organization is able to integrate clinical evidence into its day-to-day operations?

For topics that are outside the scope of this book, a list of companion readings that discuss clinical and policy issues is provided at the end of each chapter, as healthcare managers should be knowledgeable about topics that influence quality from these other perspectives as well. Although this book primarily addresses provider and delivery organizations, the concepts and approaches discussed here are also useful to managers in any healthcare-related organization (e.g., payers) or public health agency.

Managers' Perception of Quality

The healthcare researcher's perspective may dominate definitions and approaches to quality in many settings. A widely accepted definition of quality, as given by the Institute of Medicine, is "the degree to which health services for individuals and populations increase the likelihood of desired health outcomes and are consistent with current professional knowledge" (Lohr 1990).

How practicing healthcare managers define and approach quality in the context of their daily responsibilities, however, may be influenced more by their own background and experiences. For example, a physician assuming a quality management role may emphasize clinical outcomes and the implementation of evidence-based medicine or clinical practice guidelines. A statistician in that role may emphasize statistical process control and quantitative approaches. A human resources professional as a quality manager may emphasize teamwork and team-based performance appraisal, and an epidemiologist may emphasize root cause analysis. A nurse in this role may emphasize a holistic approach to quality. Likewise, a nonclinical health-care manager's educational focus can influence his or her preferred definition and approaches to quality. A manager educated in a business school may emphasize strategy, whereas someone trained as an accountant may emphasize reimbursement mechanisms. A manager with a healthcare administration background may emphasize organizational relationships and structures, and a manager educated in public health may emphasize the community.

These are just a few examples that illustrate the assortment of perspectives and preferences on quality in healthcare and the numerous ways it may be expressed within healthcare organizations. Given quality's multifaceted nature, it poses several additional questions for healthcare managers: What is quality in healthcare? Which approach is best? How are the approaches related?

According to Dalrymple and Drew (2000), "quality is conceptually complex and represents a synthesis of lessons, methods, and acquired knowledge from a range of disciplines." As a result, a healthcare manager can easily become overwhelmed by the complexity and extensive range of views on this topic. However, if the healthcare manager regards this array of perspectives as an asset rather than a barrier, he or she has the opportunity to draw from such an expanded pool of quality lessons, methods, and knowledge.

As with management practices, the subject of quality in healthcare organizations has been the object of numerous trends, fads, and attempts at quick fixes. Because departments and professionals assigned to have "quality" responsibilities may change their job titles with the latest trend, managers must understand what is being *done* in the organization to promote quality in addition to how quality-related activities are being *labeled*. The first step for managers is to develop a common understanding of quality terminology.

Definitions

This section defines and clarifies the differences among medical quality, quality assurance, continuous quality improvement, total quality, and quality management.

Medical Quality

Since the early 1970s, Avedis Donabedian's work has influenced the prevailing medical paradigm on defining and measuring quality. In his early writings, Donabedian introduced the dual nature of medical quality by describing both the technical and the interpersonal components of care (Donabedian 1980). He also identified three ways to measure quality—structure, process, and outcome measures—and the relationships among them. Donabedian described the measures in the following way (Donabedian 1980, 79, 81–83):

I have called the "process" of care . . . a set of activities that go on within and between practitioners and patients. . . . Elements of the process of care do not signify quality until their relationship to desirable health status has been established.

By "structure" I mean the relatively stable characteristics of the providers of care, of the tools and resources they have at their disposal, and of the physical and organizational settings in which they work. . . . Structure, therefore, is relevant to quality in that it increases or decreases the probability of good performance. . . .

I shall use "outcome" to mean a change in a patient's current and future health status that can be attributed to antecedent healthcare.

The fundamental functional relationship among the three elements are shown schematically as follows: Structure ➡ Process ➡ Outcome.

For example, in a multiphysician internal medicine practice, the number and credentials of physicians, physician's assistants, nurses, and office staff are considered *structure measures.* The percentage of elderly patients in this practice who appropriately received an influenza vaccine is considered a *process measure.* The percentage of elderly patients in this practice diagnosed and treated for influenza is considered an *outcome measure.* The staff in the office (structure) would influence the ability of the practice to appropriately administer the vaccine (process), which in turn would influence the number of patients developing influenza (outcome). Remember that process measures must be linked to outcomes if they are to be effective measures of quality.

Quality Assurance

A quality assurance (QA) approach involves eliminating defects. In an assembly line, defects refer to damages found in tangible products; in a service industry, like healthcare, defects refer to those performers who carry out a task or service poorly. For example, in a department that conducts insurance preauthorizations, several employees can accurately and speedily complete more preauthorizations than anyone else in the department. Alternatively, several employees, referred to as "dawdlers," can only consistently complete about half as many preauthorizations as the speedy employees. The rest of the employees are somewhere in between.

The department has certain productivity requirements or standards for the average number of preauthorizations completed per day per employee. The manager realizes that the dawdlers are dragging his productivity numbers down. He sets a minimum daily productivity level for the entire department. After several unsuccessful attempts to meet the minimum productivity goals, the workers with the poorest productivity statistics are let go. With the dawdlers gone, the department's average number of preauthorizations per employee goes up.

Figure 1.1 illustrates this manager's QA approach. The bell-shaped curve on the left, which demonstrates a normal distribution, represents the combined productivity of all of the employees in the department; it shows the result of many employees carrying out the same process over and over. A measure of central tendency is shown by the vertical line in the middle of the curve and may be represented as a mean, median, or mode (average number of preauthorizations per employee). In addition, performance varies, with a number of data points at the "better" tail of the curve (the speedy employees) and a number of data points at the "worse" tail of the curve (the dawdlers). The variation in employee outputs is represented by the width of the curve or the distance from the mean or average level of performance (the rest of the department).

The diagram on the left of the figure may be thought of as the productivity before the dawdlers are let go. This manager's QA approach is to set a threshold of performance represented by the vertical line at the worse tail of the curve (i.e., the minimum daily number of preauthorizations per employee). This threshold causes the dawdlers to stand out. When the low performance of this group is formally identified and eliminated, the average number of preauthorizations per employee increases, which is represented by the dotted vertical line to the left of the mean.

Quality Improvement

Faced with the same situation, the manager's interventions will be very different if he uses a quality improvement (QI), also referred to as continuous quality improvement (CQI), approach. The first question the manager would ask himself is, "Why are some employees really speedy and other employees take much longer to complete their work?" He talks to and observes the speedy employees first and the dawdlers next to understand how and why they take different amounts of time to do the same work. He asks the speedy people to get together, to write down the steps they go through to complete a preauthorization, and to offer any time-saving tips. The manager then calls a staff meeting so that all of the employees can learn how the speedy employees do their work. At the staff meeting, the department decides to adopt the speedy process as the new standard procedure. The speedy employees offer to train the rest of the employees in the department.

Figure 1.2 illustrates the manager's QI approach. As in the QA example, the baseline performance is represented by the bell-shaped curve on the left. However, the way in which the higher average level of performance is achieved is very different than what is seen in Figure 1.1. The

FIGURE 1.1
Quality
Assurance

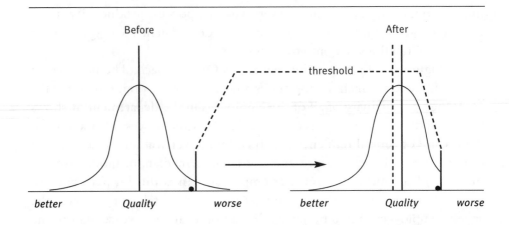

Source: Reprinted with permission from James, B. 1989. *Quality Management for Healthcare Delivery*, 37. Chicago: The Health Research and Educational Trust of the American Hospital Association.

performance resulting from improving the work process is illustrated by the shift in the entire curve to the left, which in turn raises the average level of performance. By standardizing the process used to complete a preauthorization according to the speedy employees' best practice, everyone in the office improves his or her ability to complete the preauthorizations in a more timely manner. Although there are still employees who are faster or slower, the average time to complete the preauthorization improves. In addition, the distribution is much closer to the average, which is illustrated by the narrowing of the curve; there is much less discrepancy in employee productivity than before the change is instituted. In QI, the goal is not only to improve the average performance but also to reduce inappropriate variations in the process (James 1989, 1993). In this way, the process delivers the desired output or result on a more consistent basis.

Total Quality

Because the term total quality (TQ), also referred to as total quality management (TQM), is often used interchangeably with the terms QI and CQI, students and managers may be easily confused by these two related but different concepts. The following definition clarifies the differences between TQ and CQI. Total quality is a

> philosophy or an approach to management that can be characterized by its principles, practices and techniques. Its three principles are customer focus, continuous improvement, and teamwork . . . each principle is implemented through a set of practices . . . the practices are, in turn, supported by a wide array of techniques (i.e., specific step-by-step methods intended to make the practices effective). (Dean and Bowen 1994)

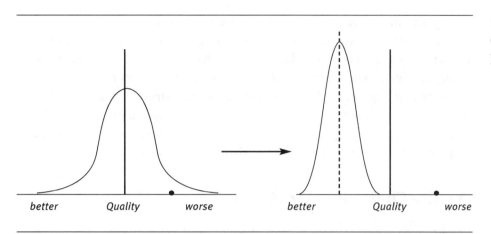

FIGURE 1.2
Quality
Improvement

Source: Reprinted with permission from James, B. 1989. *Quality Management for Healthcare Delivery*, 37. Chicago: The Health Research and Educational Trust of the American Hospital Association.

From this definition, one can see that TQ and CQI are not the same. TQ is a strategic concept, while CQI is one of three principles that support a TQ strategy. Numerous practices and techniques are available for managers to use in implementing the principle of CQI on a tactical and operational level.

Quality Management

Not only must managers understand the differences between total quality and continuous quality improvement, they must also understand the differences between quality theory and management theory. Total quality

> has evolved from a narrow focus on statistical process control to encompass a variety of technical and behavioral methods for improving organizational performance. Management theory is a multidisciplinary academic field . . . perhaps the fundamental difference between TQ and management theory is their audiences. Whereas TQ is aimed at managers, management theory is directed [at] researchers (Dean and Bowen 1994).

The overlap of these two schools of thought is referred to as organizational effectiveness, a theoretical base that not only helps the manager to improve the organization (total quality theory) but also to better understand and explain the organization (management theory) (Dean and Bowen 1994; Cole and Scott 2000).

In this book, the term "quality management" refers to the manager's role and contribution to organizational effectiveness. The book draws from management theory, quality theory as applied to non-healthcare organizations, and quality theory as applied to healthcare organizations to present practical lessons for managers and to integrate the unique characteristics of healthcare delivery and the context in which healthcare organizations operate. Quality management for our purpose refers to how managers operating in various healthcare settings (e.g., physician/manager of an individual practice, manager in a multiphysician practice, department manager in hospital, or hospital administrator) understand, explain, and improve their organizations to promote quality patient care and improve health in their communities.

Quality Continuum for Managers

Quality management does not just happen; rather, it may be viewed along a maturity continuum. Traditional or early attempts at quality represent one end of the continuum, while mature approaches to quality represent the other end. The difference between early and mature approaches to quality in healthcare organizations may be illustrated by examining how hospitals prepare for a review by the Joint Commission on Accreditation of Healthcare Organizations (JCAHO). Following are illustrations of this point.

Hospital A is a large academic medical center. More than 12 years ago, its chief executive officer (CEO) demonstrated his support for quality by changing the QA department to the CQI department and hiring a director of CQI. The JCAHO coordinator and the CQI coordinator report to the CQI director. The three staff members who report to the JCAHO coordinator are responsible for hospital accreditation preparation and for collecting and reporting the performance measures required by JCAHO. The five staff members who report to the CQI coordinator assist teams throughout the hospital with improvement projects by providing facilitation, teaching improvement tools, and collecting and reporting data on the improvements.

Hospital A goes through the JCAHO review every three years, and the review preparation process has been the same for as long as anyone can remember. Nine months before the review, a master task list is developed by the JCAHO coordinator. The coordinator and/or her staff meet with every department manager to give out assignments and the timeline for completion. At the monthly hospital manager's meeting, the coordinator provides a progress report and announces the "countdown until Joint Commission." Three months prior to the review, the coordinator's staff works six days a week. The last month prior to the review, the CQI staff typically works 12 hours a day, six days a week. The level of stress in the organization gradually increases over the nine months of preparation, and the organization is in a state of frenzy a few weeks before the review. The surveyors arrive. The review is successfully completed, and the hospital even receives high praise for two of the CQI presentations the CQI coordinator prepared.

Hospital B is also a large academic medical center. Until ten years ago, the hospital approached the JCAHO review process in a manner similar to that of Hospital A. At that time, a new CEO was just hired, and as he was getting acquainted with managers throughout the hospital, he asked a simple question: "What would happen if we operated every day as if the Joint Commission were coming?" Systematically, he began to create an organizational culture that he believed would be the answer to his question.

Hospital B also had two, separate quality department groups: one group was focused on accreditation and one group was involved in facilitating CQI projects. The first thing the new CEO did was merge the two groups into one and rename the department as the quality resources department. Rather than make the quality resources department the entity solely responsible for quality-related activities in the hospital, the CEO redefined the role of every manager throughout the hospital to include expectations for performance results, improvement projects, and JCAHO accreditation. Each manager was assigned a dedicated quality consultant from the quality resources department who would serve as a resource on measurement; data collection and analysis; JCAHO standards; and improvement tools, methods, and facilitation. Some quality consultants supported many small units, while some quality consultants supported a few large units.

The CEO also set new expectations for the administrators who reported to him. With his administrative team, he began to review monthly reports on patient satisfaction, financial performance, clinical outcomes, and productivity. As a group, they reviewed trends and discussed performance-related issues. After a year, the CEO asked the administrators to set their own performance goals based on opportunities identified from these monthly performance discussions. In turn, the administrators worked with the managers who reported to them to set department-level goals that were consistent with the administrative-level performance goals. All department managers were involved. For example, the pharmacy manager set the goal to improve the time to fill an outpatient prescription, while the finance manager set the goal to design financial reports that were more useful to managers.

The CEO also redesigned the hospital newsletter to include a "CEO Update" column that reported the hospital's performance and any business or market issues affecting the hospital. Finally, the CEO dug out employee satisfaction survey results from the last several years. He studied them as part of setting his own goals to address sources of employee dissatisfaction. He considered it his responsibility to create the culture and to provide the environment, resources, and tools that would best enable employees to deliver quality care to patients.

As the JCAHO review date approaches for Hospital B, announcements are made and final details are addressed. The week of the surveyors' visit is seen as "business as usual." The survey is successfully completed without much stress.

Hospital A exemplifies a traditional or less mature approach to quality. The focus is on meeting standards and eliminating defects. Quality is the job of specialists, while responsibilities for both JCAHO and continuous improvement belong to the CQI department. Progress along the continuum is seen when the hospital adopts CQI techniques to improve work processes. This point is demonstrated by the CQI projects sponsored by Hospital A's CQI department staff.

Hospital B exemplifies an organization that is progressing to a more mature state along the quality continuum. Hospital leaders demonstrate quality through their actions and through the direction they set for the organization. Quality is the responsibility of everyone in the organization rather than something that is delegated to specialists. Requirements of both internal and external customers and stakeholders are recognized and addressed. All processes—both clinical patient care processes and internal operational and administrative processes—in the organization are targeted for improvement. Ongoing measurement and understanding of past and current performance support the organization's ability to continually improve its results for patients and other stakeholders.

Although a healthcare organization may occupy a point anywhere along this maturity continuum, the goal of quality management is to continually strive toward the most mature end of the continuum. Figure 1.3 illustrates how the continuum may be viewed for healthcare organizations.

Conclusion

By understanding the quality continuum in healthcare, managers can begin to see

- how an organization can be successful at CQI projects but not at attaining a quality organizational culture;
- why defining clinical practice guidelines does not in itself guarantee healthcare quality;
- why organizational development efforts, independent of clinical context, may not yield expected results; and
- why, without leadership's involvement in establishing a quality philosophy for the entire organization, only pockets of excellence may be found throughout the organization.

The rest of Section I provides a more in-depth discussion of total quality, beginning with the three principles of customer focus, continuous improvement, and teamwork in Chapter 2. The remainder of this book focuses on quality management by providing healthcare managers with practical lessons to assist them in their journey along the quality continuum.

• Meet standards
• Eliminate defects
	• Products:
	  Healthcare
	  delivery
		• Products: All products,
		  goods, and services,
		  whether for sale or not—
		  care delivery, public
		  healthcare, payers,
		  equipment, supplies	

	• Processes:
	  Clinical
	  procedures/
	  support
	  processes
		• Processes: All processes
		  —clinical, business,
		  operational, support,
		  manufacturing, decision
		  making, policy	

	• Customers:
	  Patients,
	  physicians
	• Clients who buy
	  the products:
	  Patients, payers
		• Customers and other
		  stakeholders: Anyone who
		  has an expectation of, is
		  interested in, or is affected
		  by the work of the
		  organization—patients,
		  families, internal customers
		  employers, communities,
		  organizations, regulators	

	• Cost of poor quality:
	  Financial
		• Costs of poor quality: All
		  costs that would disappear
		  if everything were perfect
		  —financial, quality of life,
		  productivity, opportunity
		  costs	

Less Mature		**More Mature**	

FIGURE 1.3
Quality
Continuum
for Healthcare
Managers

Source: Adapted from Juran, J. M. 1989. *Juran on Leadership for Quality: An Executive Handbook*, 48. New York: The Free Press.

Companion Readings

Brook, R., H. E. McGlynn, and P. G. Shekell. 2000. "Defining and Measuring Quality of Care: A Perspective from US Researchers." *International Journal for Quality in Healthcare* 12 (4): 281–95.

Institute of Medicine. 2001. *Crossing the Quality Chasm: A New Health System for the 21st Century,* 1–38. Washington, DC: National Academy Press.

Mullan, F. 2001. "A Founder of Quality Assessment Encounters a Troubled System Firsthand." *Health Affairs* 20 (1): 137–41.

References

Cole, R. E., and W. R. Scott, eds. 2000. *The Quality Movement and Organization Theory.* Thousand Oaks, CA: Sage Publications.

Dalrymple, J., and E. Drew. 2000. "Quality: On the Threshold or the Brink?" *Total Quality Management* 11 (4/5 & 6): 697–703.

Dean, J. W., and D. E. Bowen. 1994. "Management Theory and Total Quality: Improving Research and Practice through Theory Development." *Academy of Management Review* 19 (2): 392–418.

Donabedian, A. 1980. *Explorations in Quality Assessment and Monitoring, Volume I: The Definition of Quality and Approaches to Its Assessment.* Chicago: Health Administration Press.

James, B. 1993. "Implementing Practice Guidelines Through Clinical Quality Improvement." *Frontiers of Health Services Management* 10 (1): 3–37.

———. 1989. *Quality Management for Healthcare Delivery.* Chicago: The Health Research and Educational Trust of the American Hospital Association.

Juran, J. M. 1989. *Juran on Leadership for Quality: An Executive Handbook,* 48. New York: The Free Press.

Lohr, K. N. 1990. *Medicare: A Strategy for Quality Assurance.* Washington, DC: National Academy Press.

Exercise

Objective: To explore how managers influence the quality of products, services, and the customer experience

Instructions:

1. Think of an experience where you received or observed excellent quality. This experience may have been as a customer, as a patient, as a provider, or as an employee. Describe the factors that made this an excellent experience and how you felt as a result of this experience. Include a description of management's influence on your experience. Do the same for a situation in which you experienced poor quality. Record your responses in the table below or one similar to it.

	Briefly describe the experience.	Describe what made this an excellent or poor quality experience.	How did you feel as a result?	What was management's role or influence?
Excellent Quality				
Poor Quality				

2. On the basis of your observations above, describe why it is important for healthcare managers to understand quality.

THREE PRINCIPLES OF TOTAL QUALITY

Objectives

- To describe the three principles of total quality: customer focus, continuous improvement, and teamwork
- To begin to explore how these three principles may be expressed in the managerial role
- To practice identifying management behaviors that demonstrate these three principles

Any healthcare manager would probably say that quality patient care, quality outcomes, or health improvement factored into their decision to pursue a career in healthcare. However, translating a commitment to quality into management actions and interactions has remained elusive to managers. The previous chapter defined total quality as "a philosophy or an approach to management that can be characterized by its principles, practices, and techniques. Its three principles are customer focus, continuous improvement, and teamwork" (Dean and Bowen 1994). In this chapter, we begin to explore how managers may strategically integrate the principles of total quality into how they carry out managerial functions.

The information presented in this chapter is not intended to replace management knowledge and skills in areas such as finance, human resources, strategy, or marketing; rather, this information should complement those areas. By viewing their role through a total quality lens, managers may enhance their overall ability to use their range of knowledge. By doing this, they will be better able to achieve desired results within their scope of responsibility, whether for an entire organization, a department, or a team.

Principle 1: Customer Focus

The principle of customer focus may be better applied when the manager is aware of the dual nature of medical quality and is able to define customers and stakeholders as well as their respective expectations and requirements.

Dual Nature of Quality

Managers must remember that many clinical healthcare professionals have been educated from a philosophy that defines quality according to the professionals' expertise and expectations rather than according to the patient's or customer's expectations or requirements. In Chapter 1, the dual nature of medical quality as described by Donabedian (technical and interpersonal components of care) was introduced. The term *content quality* refers to clinical expertise and technical aspects of healthcare (e.g., diagnosing an illness correctly or carrying out a clinical procedure properly). Most patients assume that providers possess and deliver technical quality. The terms *delivery quality* and *service quality* refer to the interpersonal components of care (e.g., empathy and communication) and to how well the patients' requirements and expectations are being met (e.g., access, timely billing) (James 1989).

To manage from a total quality philosophy, managers should first determine the extent they themselves, providers, and other employees understand and accept the dual nature of quality. Managers, as department or organizational leaders, are responsible for establishing a customer-focused environment and direction for their employees. This comment from a skilled technical nurse—"I wish the family would get out of the way so I could do my job"—suggests a work environment in which content quality is valued and rewarded above service quality. Policies and procedures, job descriptions, personnel performance expectations and evaluations, reward systems, and staff development may be viewed as tools to aid the manager in creating a customer-focused environment. By purposefully and strategically incorporating both aspects of quality care into the design of these management tools, managers may enhance their ability to implement a focus on both content and service quality.

Defining Customers and Stakeholders

A customer is anyone who has an expectation about the output of a process (James 1989). *External customers* are those parties outside of the organization. Healthcare organizations regard patients, families, and significant others as their primary external customers.

The customer focus principle requires managers who are operating from a total quality philosophy to not only be attentive to their external customers but also to their internal customers and stakeholders. An *internal customer* comes from within the organization. This type of customer may be someone who is responsible for activities that are "downstream" from the ones somebody else is doing. For example, in a hospital, when patient care is handed off from one provider to another at shift change, the incoming provider is considered the internal customer of the outgoing provider. Completing the requisite shift responsibilities in a timely manner and leaving a tidy work space demonstrate a recognition of coworkers as internal customers.

Anyone with an interest in or who is affected by the work of an individual, a department, or an organization is referred to as a *stakeholder*. In healthcare organizations, stakeholders may include "the community, insurers/third-party payors, employers, health care providers, patient advocacy groups, [and] Departments of Health" (National Institutes for Standards and Technology 2002). Defining customers and stakeholders is a prerequisite to determining their requirements.

Customer Requirements

In addition to behaviors, such as courtesy, at the interpersonal level, operating from a customer-focused position requires an understanding not only of who the customers are but also of what these customers require; how the requirements differ between customer groups; how these requirements change over time; and how these requirements guide organizational strategy, decisions, and activities (National Institute for Standards and Technology 2002). The advent of evening outpatient clinic hours illustrates how organizational decisions on hours of operation have changed to keep pace with changing patient work schedules and employment requirements.

Patients as customer groups may be differentiated by disease category (e.g., cancer, cardiovascular, obstetrics), age, the nature of the illness (e.g., chronic, acute), the site of care (e.g., inpatient, outpatient, long-term care), ethnicity, or language. The federal government is an example of a key stakeholder and one that has demonstrated changing requirements over the past several years, particularly in the area of quality reporting (Jencks et al. 2000; James 1993). An understanding of both patient requirements and federal government requirements should factor into how managers design performance measurement systems.

Principle 2: Continuous Improvement

The principle of continuous improvement may be expressed through a manager's day-to-day actions, managerial functions, and support for improvement projects.

Day-to-Day Actions

It is not uncommon for the manager of the environmental services department in a large hospital to pick up something from the hallway floor and throw it away in the nearest trash can. This manager's action exemplifies the principle of continuous improvement. While other hospital employees would walk past or over the trash, this environmental services manager realizes the importance of being committed to continuous improvement for his or her department and for the hospital; if at any time he or she saw something that needed fixing, improving, or correcting, he or she would take the initiative. If managers want to achieve continuous improvement in their organizations, they must demonstrate continuous improvement through their everyday actions.

Managerial Functions

The principle of continuous improvement may also be expressed through managers' execution of their managerial functions. For example, managers operating from this principle consider a performance measurement system an essential tool. This system includes indicators reported at various time intervals, depending on the nature of the work and the scope of management responsibility. For example, a shift supervisor for the patient transportation service in an 800-bed academic medical center watches the electronic dispatch system that displays a minute-by-minute update on transportation requests, indicators of patients en route to their destination, and the number of patients in the queue. By monitoring the system, the supervisor is immediately aware if a problem occurs and, as a result, is quickly able to take action to resolve the problem. If the number of requests unexpectedly increases, the supervisor can reassign staff breaks to maximize staff availability and minimize response times.

Each day, the supervisor posts the total number of transports performed the previous day along with the average response times. This way, the patient transporters are aware of the department's statistics and their own individual statistics, and this helps the transporters take pride in a job that is typically underappreciated by others in the organization. The daily performance data also enable the supervisor to quickly identify and address documented complaints and to address them within 24 hours, which in turn increases employee accountability and improves customer relations. On a monthly basis, the department manager and the shift supervisors review the volume of requests by hour of the day to determine if employees are scheduled appropriately to meet demand. The manager also reviews the statistics sorted by patient unit (e.g., nursing unit, radiology department) to identify any issues that need to be explored directly, manager to manager. The monthly statistics are reviewed by the manager with the administrator to whom the manager reports, while the annual statistics are used in the budgeting process.

A performance measurement and management system such as this enables managers to continually monitor performance; to identify quality issues and performance gaps and to take action to resolve them; and to provide a foundation for ongoing communication, planning, and accountability.

Support for an Improvement Project

Continuous improvement may also be expressed when managers support continuous quality improvement projects that address specific problems or performance gaps. An improvement project involves assembling a team to solve a problem or improve performance in a designated area. The team is responsible for designing and implementing improvements to the underlying work process. Managers may demonstrate their support of project teams by effectively initiating the project, promoting buy-in, and taking specific management actions that will help the team succeed.

Initiating a Project

Managers should attend to three areas when initiating an improvement project: define participant accountabilities, establish boundaries, and communicate managerial expectations.

First, the accountabilities of all participants should be clearly defined. Accountabilities may include how decisions will be made or what type of participation is expected from members of the team (e.g., attendance). Defining accountabilities does not necessarily mean that the manager makes all the rules; rather, he or she ensures that the rules are clearly defined. For example, when the administrator asked the surgeons how they would like to be involved in an upcoming improvement effort to address patient flow in the preoperative area, the surgeons indicated that they would prefer to have a proposed plan presented to them at their monthly medical staff meetings. They would then provide feedback and recommendations during their already established governance structure. They did not have the time or desire to be involved in the day-to-day details of designing the improvements, but they definitely wanted to be part of the process of evaluating and refining proposed solutions.

Managers should clearly define the boundaries of what can and cannot be changed—that is, what aspects of the problem, solution, or process are negotiable and not negotiable. For example, the improvement team of an emergency department was told to think "outside the box." However, when the team presented its "outside the box" and very expensive idea to hospital administration, the team was told that the idea was impossible to implement because of the associated expense. The lack of boundaries, rather than spurring creativity, ended up demoralizing the team members and discouraging them from continuing to participate in this or future improvement efforts. The morale and engagement of the team members could have been preserved had the manager defined the boundaries for the team, such as the maximum dollars available for remodeling or new equipment, very early in the improvement effort.

Finally, if an improvement team needs to deliver specific results or follow specific constraints, these expectations should be clearly defined and communicated at the onset of any change or improvement effort. Expectations may include timelines (e.g., within a certain operating budget cycle), results (e.g., improve cycle times by 5 percent), or budgets (e.g., dollars or time allotted for project team meetings).

Promoting Buy-In

To promote staff buy-in, the manager should "sell the problem, not the solution" (Bridges 1991). When employees are informed about the nature and consequences of the problem, they are much more likely to be open to various solutions designed to improve it.

Managers should also be careful to build on the current strengths and accomplishments of their staff. If not introduced tactfully, an improvement effort may send the unintended message that employees are not doing a good job. For example, a manager began a new position at a state health department after working for many years in a hospital that had been recognized for its quality-improvement efforts. This manager had been recruited to help the health department improve its work processes to become more efficient. As the manager became acquainted with the department, she realized that the focus on efficiency was a response to major budget cuts in the recent legislative session. As she introduced her goals of improved efficiency to employees in the department, she first acknowledged the successful programs that the department had designed and implemented. She then educated the employees about specific changes in the environment and stakeholder requirements. To respond to these changing external factors, the department needed to evaluate and adapt its internal operations. Next, she explained that to preserve funds for the department programs, the department needed to become more efficient and productive in how they administered these programs.

Helping the Team Succeed

For a project team to be effective, it must have a clear understanding of what it has been organized to do. The manager must provide clear direction for the team; techniques for setting goals will be further described in Chapter 7.

The manager should also provide the opportunity for team members to interact with each other and others in the organization. When thinking about the composition of a project team, participants from outside of the manager's own scope of responsibility should be considered if they have fundamental knowledge of the process targeted for improvement. For example, a team organized to improve discharge planning in an inpatient surgical unit in a large hospital included not only nurses from this unit but from "upstream care" (i.e., operating room and intensive care unit) and non-nursing providers (i.e., dietician, social worker, and respiratory therapist). In this way the team integrated all of the aspects and sources of care the patients received during their hospital stay into the discharge planning process.

The manager is instrumental in ensuring access to the information that the team needs to effectively study and improve the problem. Information may come in many forms such as management reports, clinical data, and regulatory requirements. Managers may also assist teams by providing access to information that the team may not know is available. For example, one manager helped a team organize a discussion with several internal customers so that they could better understand their customers' perspective. Another manager helped link a team with the organization's corporate marketing department, which in turn invited the team members to observe a patient focus group. This manager also helped the team to schedule the hospital administrator to come to one of their meetings to answer questions and address concerns.

Principle 3: Teamwork

In many organizations, when the terms "teamwork" and "quality" are used together, they usually refer to cross-functional or interdisciplinary project teams. The principle of teamwork may also be thought of in relation to philosophies and approaches used in carrying out the numerous functions inherent in the managerial role.

Management Philosophy

In the old days, when a physician entered the hospital unit, nurses were accustomed to offering their chairs to the physician because the nurses held lower positions in the organizational and professional hierarchy. Remnants of this tradition (i.e., deferring to someone higher in the hierarchy, ordering about someone lower in the hierarchy) may still be seen in healthcare organizations that operate from a bureaucratic philosophy.

An academic medical center, for example, may operate from a bureaucratic philosophy represented by multiple and parallel hierarchies. The CEO and the administrative team occupy the top positions in the management hierarchy, while frontline supervisors occupy the bottom. The department chairs are at the top of the medical staff hierarchy, and the interns or medical students are at the bottom. Physicians, followed by nurses, are at the top of the professional hierarchy, while other professionals (e.g., social workers, occupational therapists) all hold nondescript places lower in the hierarchy. Physicians and nurses hold the top spots in the jobs hierarchy, while the hourly manual laborers (e.g., environmental services and food service workers) are designated to the lower spots.

Although each group performs its respective duties in a competent manner, a lack of coordination among the groups and a lack of a common patient care approach can be observed. For example, physician teams typically make their morning patient rounds while nurses are occupied with the change-of-shift report. As a result, the nurses and physicians caring for the same patients rarely talk to each other during the course of day-to-day patient care.

Another example of this lack of coordination is that although a hospital can demonstrate many examples of continuous quality improvement team projects, its teams tend to have an exclusive make up (i.e., physician teams or nurse teams). Even though departments, such as the laboratory, have attempted on numerous occasions to create improvement teams with a mix of different providers, they have had little success in crossing the rigid boundaries of the professional and job hierarchies in the organization. Although a hospital is able to identify many teams, only a few examples of teamwork across and within these hierarchies can be seen.

Management Functions

The manner by which management functions are implemented may promote or unintentionally discourage teamwork within the organization. The relationship between teamwork and three managerial functions—organizational design, resource allocation, and communication—is discussed in this section.

Organizational Design

Organizational design has been identified as a critical management function (Shortell and Kaluzny 2000). Some organizational designs, such as a matrix structure or a service-line structure, may promote teamwork. A *matrix structure* is characterized by a dual authority system. In a *service-line structure,* a single person is responsible for all aspects of a group of services, usually based on patient type (e.g., pediatric, women's services, oncology, transplant services) (Shortell and Kaluzny 2000).

One large hospital used a hybrid of these two structures in its approach to organizational design. Each administrator had responsibility for multiple departments that cared for patients with similar needs. For example, the trauma administrator was responsible for the emergency department, the trauma intensive care unit, and the air transport service. Although finance, human resources, and quality resources operated from their own centralized departments to maintain his or her unique competencies, each administrator in the hospital was assigned his or her own finance, human resources, and quality "consultants." Teamwork between the administrators and the dedicated staff consultants enhanced the ability of the staff to provide consistent and responsive service to both the administrators and the managers for whom they were responsible.

Resource Allocation

A large acute care hospital was organized according to a functional design where "labor is divided into departments specialized by functional area" (Shortell and Kaluzny 2000). Although teamwork across functions in daily patient care may be difficult, it is not impossible, a point illustrated by one resourceful supervisor.

A centralized respiratory therapy department provided services for all of the intensive care units and the inpatient units. The respiratory therapists usually rotated among units and rarely worked more than a couple of days in a row on the same one. One supervisor was able to promote teamwork between nurses and respiratory therapists through strategic staff scheduling and assignments.

In this facility, although the majority of patients were adults, the women's services included a labor and delivery unit and a neonatal intensive care unit. The knowledge and skills needed by the respiratory therapists to care for the neonates were very different from the knowledge and skills they needed to care for adults. Maintaining a current level of competency required the respiratory therapists to work consistently and frequently on the neonatal intensive care unit.

To address this need, the supervisor designed a core team of respiratory therapists dedicated to staffing the neonatal intensive care unit. The therapists continued to report to her as the respiratory therapy supervisor. Because the therapists were only assigned to one unit (except on rare occasions), they not only maintained their clinical expertise with the neonatal population, they were able to develop trust and ongoing working relationships with the unit nurses, which in turn fostered teamwork in daily patient care delivery.

Communication

The principle of teamwork may also be reflected in the way managers design communication processes and structures. In one hospital, the manager of the materials management department negotiated with a supplier to obtain surgical gloves at a discounted rate, compared to the rate of the current supplier; the decision was made based on vendor and financial input. The first time the new gloves were used, the surgeon ripped out the fingers of the gloves while inserting his hand.

Had the manager embraced the concept of teamwork in his approach to decision making, he would have sought out information and input from the patient care team—the people who actually used the product and knew the advantages and disadvantages of different brands of gloves.

Conclusion

This chapter begins our exploration of how the three principles of total quality—customer focus, continuous improvement, and teamwork—influence the way managers carry out their respective roles and functions. Although the examples provided in this chapter only begin to mention the implications for managers, the examples raise managers' awareness that their decisions and actions affect their ability to implement these principles throughout their entire organizations. Readers are encouraged to continuously question how they can integrate the principles of total quality into decisions and activities inherent in their roles as managers. The exercise at the end of this chapter is designed to assist the reader to identify additional management behaviors and approaches that express the three principles of total quality. An overview of tools commonly used to implement the principle of continuous quality improvement is presented in Chapter 3.

Companion Readings

Morton, J. 1995. "Improving Customer Satisfaction: Emerging Lessons About Strategy and Implementation." *Managed Care Quarterly* 3 (2): 33–42.

————. 1995. "Improving Customer Satisfaction: Emerging Lessons About Strategy and Implementation, Part 2." *Managed Care Quarterly* 3 (3): 30–45.

References

Bridges, W. 1991. *Managing Transitions: Making the Most of Change.* Reading, MA: Addison Publishing Company.

Dean, J. W., and D. E. Bowen. 1994. "Management Theory and Total Quality: Improving Research and Practice through Theory Development." *Academy of Management Review* 19 (2): 392–418.

James, B. 1993. "Implementing Practice Guidelines through Clinical Quality Improvement." *Frontiers of Health Services Management* 10 (1): 3–37.

————. 1989. *Quality Management for Healthcare Delivery.* Chicago: The Health Research and Educational Trust of the American Hospital Association.

Jencks, S. F., T. Cuerdon, D. R. Burwen, B. Fleming, P. M. Houck, A. E. Kussmaul, D. S. Nilasena, D. L. Ordin, and D. R. Arday. 2000. "Quality of Medical Care Delivered to Medicare Beneficiaries: A Profile at State and National Levels." *Journal of the American Medical Association* 284 (13): 1670–76.

National Institute for Standards and Technology. 2002. *Healthcare Criteria for Performance Excellence.* Washington, DC: National Institute for Standards and Technology.

Shortell, S. M., and A. D. Kaluzny. 2000. *Healthcare Management: Organization Design and Behavior.* Albany, NY: Delmar Thomson Learning.

Exercise

Objective: Practice identifying management behaviors that express the three principles of total quality: customer focus, continuous improvement, and teamwork.

Instructions:

The following account of an improvement effort in an ambulatory surgery unit is told by the former *Wall Street Journal* columnist Thomas Petzinger, Jr.

1.   Read the case study.
2.   Describe at least one example of how management in this case study demonstrated the principle of customer focus.
3.   Describe at least one example of how management in this case study demonstrated the principle of continuous improvement.
4.   Describe at least one example of how management in this case study demonstrated the principle of teamwork.

Case Study

This case study is excerpted with permission of Simon & Schuster Adult Publishing Group from *The New Pioneers: The Men and Women Who Are Transforming the Workplace and the Marketplace* by Thomas Petzinger, Jr. Copyright © 1999 by Thomas Petzinger, Jr.

While many companies are getting better at customer service, one industry has gotten a lot worse lately. That industry is medicine. The onslaught of managed care has commoditized what was once the most delicate relationship in all of commerce, that of doctor and patient. The practice of "capitation" creates the risk of a doctor visit becoming a cattle call. Accounting for the payment of services has overwhelmed the rendering of the services themselves. Yet a few islands of people have thrown off their Newtonian blinders and recognized that putting the customer first can redound to the benefit of the provider as well. With so many competing claims on every dollar, every process, and every hour of time and attention, the interests of the customer—the patient—serve as a common ground for making the entire system more efficient.

One hospital is such a place: a 520-bed teaching hospital and so-called trauma-one center with a stellar clinical reputation. Within the hospital, an outpatient surgery clinic was opened long ago, in which an ever-larger percentage of procedures were being conducted. And although the surgical staff was acclaimed, management recognized that the overall patient experience left something to be desired.

The main problem was delay. The surgery line was jam-packed as early as 5:30 every morning. Some patients spent the entire day lurching from check-in to pre-op to anesthesia to surgery to recovery to post-op, with too much of the time spent simply waiting. As much as some people may wish to convalesce at length as admitted hospital patients, no one wants to turn a four-hour outpatient experience into a nine-hour ordeal. If the hospital wanted to maintain (much less extend) its position in the marketplace, it had to figure out how to get patients through faster without degrading clinical results.

The job of facilitating the planning process went to an internal quality consultant who had worked for fifteen years as a registered nurse, mostly in neonatal intensive care, before earning her MBA and fulfilling this new organizational role. In her years in intensive care, she was often perplexed by the priorities that families exhibited in even the most dire medical situations. "I'm working like crazy to save a baby, but the parents get upset because the grandparents didn't get to see the baby!" she recalls. In time she could see that medicine was only part of health care. "Health care providers hold people's lives in their hands at a very vulnerable time," she says. "Health care is about a personal encounter." Most of the people on the business side of health care have little intellectual grasp and even less emotional grasp of this concept. Indeed, after moving to the business side herself, she became convinced that some of the most intractable problems of the industry could be solved only by people who, like her, combined far-flung disciplines. "Innovation will come from people who have crossed the boundaries from other disciplines," she says—from business to medicine, from medicine to law, and so on.

The facilitator insisted on involving the maximum number of nurses—people . . . who knew the whole patient as well as the individual surgeries they variously received. The new administrator over the area requested that the members of the improvement committee visit as many other hospitals as possible, within their large hospital system, to explore which outpatient surgical practices could be employed at their own site. And throughout the study process, the administrator continually harped on the "vision statement" of the initiative, which put as its first priority "to provide a patient/family focused quality culture."

This new administrator in the surgery service, a nurse herself, was a powerful force in leading the improvement effort. Under the previous leadership, the policy for change was simply "give the surgeons whatever they want," as she put it. The administrator acknowledged that the surgeon must call the shots on procedures—but not necessarily on process. In that respect she, too, insisted on using the patient as the point of departure. "If you're guided by only one phrase—what is best for the patient—you will always come up with the right answer," the administrator insists. (Hearing the administrator and facilitator say this over and over began to remind me of the best editors I have worked for. When in doubt, they would often say, do only what's right for the reader. Everything else will fall into place.)

Studying the surgery line from the patients' point of view was disturbingly illuminating. Surgeons showing up late for the first round of surgeries at 7:30 a.m. threw off the schedule for the entire day. The various hospital departments—admitting, financing, lab, surgery—all conducted their own separate interaction with the patient on each of their individual schedules. A poor physical layout, including a long corridor separating the operating rooms from pre-op, compounded the inefficiencies. Once a patient was called to surgery, he spent forty minutes waiting for an orderly to arrive with a wheelchair or gurney. And, because this was an outpatient surgery center located inside a hospital, the anesthesiologists were accustomed to administering heavy sedation, often slowing the patient's recovery from otherwise minor surgery and further clogging the entire line. The operation was a success, but the patient was pissed.

In talking to patients, the researchers discovered a subtext in the complaints about delays: resentment over the loss of personal control. Patients spent the day in God-awful gauze gowns, stripped of their underwear, their backsides exposed to the world. Partly this reflected a medical culture that considered the procedure, not the patient, as the customer. As the administrator put it to me, "If you're naked on a stretcher on your back, you're pretty subservient." Family members, meanwhile, had to roam the hospital in search of change so they could coax a cup of coffee from a vending machine. She marveled at the arrogance of it. "You're spending $3,000 on a loved one, but you'd better bring correct change."

Fortunately, this administrator had the political standing to push through big changes, and although the staff surgeons effectively had veto power, most were too busy to get very deeply involved in the improvement process. Because few patients enjoy getting stuck with needles, the nurses created a process for capturing the blood from the insertion of each patient's intravenous needle and sending it to the lab for whatever tests were necessary. This cut down not only on discomfort, but on time, money and scheduling complexity. The unremitting bureaucratic questions and paperwork were all replaced with a single registration packet that patients picked up in their doctors' offices and completed days before ever setting foot in the hospital; last-minute administrative details were attended to in a single phone call the day before surgery. The nurses set up a check-in system for the coats and valuables of patients and family members, which eliminated the need for every family to encamp with their belongings in a pre-op room for the entire day. A family-friendly waiting area was created, stocked with free snacks and drinks. There would be no more desperate searches for correct change.

That was only the beginning. Patients had always resented having to purchase their post-op medications from the hospital pharmacy; simply freeing them to use their neighborhood drugstore got them out of the surgery line sooner, further relieving the congestion. Also in the interests of saving time, the nurses made a heretical proposal to allow healthy outpatients to walk into surgery under their own power, accompanied by their family members, rather than waiting forty minutes for a wheelchair of gurney. That idea got the attention of the surgeons, who after years of paying ghastly malpractice premiums vowed that the administrator, not they, would suffer the personal liability on that one. The risk-management department went "eek" at the idea. Yet as the improvement committee pointed out, the hospital permitted outpatients to traverse any other distance in the building by foot. Why should the march into surgery be any different?

In a similar vein, the nurses suggested allowing patients to wear underwear beneath their hospital gowns. The administrators could scarcely believe their ears: "Show me one place in the literature where patients wear underwear to surgery!" one top administrator demanded. (The nurses noted that restricting change to what had been attempted elsewhere would automatically eliminate the possibility of any breakthrough in performance.) And why stop at underwear, the nurses asked? The hospital was conducting more and more outpatient cataract operations; why not let these patients wear their clothes into surgery? "Contamination!" the purists cried. But clothing is no dirtier than the skin beneath it, the nurses answered. This change eliminated a major post-op bottleneck caused by elderly patients who could not dress themselves or tie their shoes with their heads clouded by anesthesia and their depth perception altered by the removal of their cataracts.

As the changes took effect, the nurses observed another unintended effect. Patients were actually reducing their recovery times! People were no longer looking at ceiling tiles on their way into surgery like characters in an episode of *Dr. Kildare.* They went into surgery feeling better and came out of it feeling better. In case after case they were ready to leave the joint faster, which in turn freed up even more space for other patients. Because they had studied practices at a number of stand-alone clinics, the nurses even suggested to the physicians that the outpatients would be better off with less anesthesia, hastening their recoveries, speeding their exit, and freeing up still more capacity.

Within a year, the volume at the outpatient surgery unit had surged 50 percent with no increase in square footage and no increase in staff. Customer-service surveys were positive and costs were under control. And it dawned on the facilitator that the nurses' intuitive conviction that the patient should come first benefited the surgery line itself at every single step. Everyone and everything connected to the process—surgeon, staff, insurers, time, cost, and quality—seemed to come out ahead when the patients' interests came first.

What was really happening, of course, was that the change teams simply put common sense first. In a complex process of many players, the interest of the patient was the one unifying characteristic—the best baseline for calibration—because the patient was the only person touched by every step.

3

CONTINUOUS QUALITY IMPROVEMENT TOOLS

Objectives

* To introduce commonly used continuous improvement tools
* To practice using the continuous improvement tools

An employee was faced with choosing a new primary care physician when her employer changed health plans. This employee made a list of the characteristics she wanted in a physician (e.g., board certified) and in the physician's office (e.g., close to work). She asked fellow employees and friends if they knew any of the physicians listed in the health plan handbook and what they thought of their care experiences. She then selected a physician and made an appointment for an annual physical. After her first experience with the new physician, she decided that both the physician and the office staff met her criteria and that she would continue to use the physician as her primary care doctor.

Although this employee may not have realized it, the continuous-improvement approach used in her organization had "rubbed off" on her so that she automatically used the same systematic process for deciding what to do when faced with a personal problem or decision. She planned how to select a physician; compared the various options against her criteria; tested her first choice; and, based on her impressions and experiences, decided to keep her first choice as her primary care physician. She had used a variation of what is referred to in the quality improvement literature as the Shewhart Cycle (Figure 3.1).

Originating from industrial applications of quality improvement, the *Shewhart Cycle* (also referred to as the PDCA Cycle) consists of four steps: planning, doing, checking/studying, and acting. The steps are linked to represent the cyclical nature of the approach. In the planning step, the process of concern is investigated and studied to better understand the problem(s) and to identify how to improve the process. In the doing step, the new process or intervention is implemented on a small scale to test its effectiveness. The checking/studying step involves monitoring the results of the intervention to determine how well the new process is working. Finally, in the acting step, the results and effects are reviewed to determine what was learned from the small-scale trial. On the basis of what was learned

FIGURE 3.1

Shewhart
Cycle

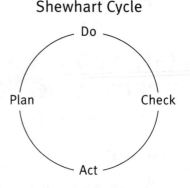

Shewhart Cycle

1. Plan → study the process
2. Do → make the change on a small scale
3. Check → observe the effects
4. Act → identify what was learned

Cycle is ongoing and continuous

Source: Walton, M. 1986. *The Deming Management Method,* 86. New York: The Putnam Publishing Group.

from the test, the new process is studied and refinements are made, and this second planning step begins the cycle again.

Often an organization may select and endorse a particular improvement technique, such as the Shewhart Cycle, found in the quality improvement literature (Institute for Healthcare Improvement 2003; Juran 1989; Langley et al. 1996; Scholtes, Joiner, and Streibel 1996; Walton 1986). Managers will find that the common elements in these techniques are that they include systematically identifying causes of problems, designing and implementing improvements, and monitoring and continually improving the effects of the intervention. The tools presented in this chapter will assist managers as they approach continuous improvement within the context of their own organization's preferred technique.

Improvement Tools

CQI tools focus a team's problem-solving efforts and provide a document trail that managers may use to organize and record the improvement process and results of the project. Documentation is essential to ensure continuity between project meetings and to provide a mechanism for sharing knowledge, ongoing learning, encouraging follow-up on outcomes, and building team confidence through a concrete display of the team's accomplishments.

Improvement tools fall into four general categories:

1. identifying customer expectations,
2. documenting a process,
3. diagnosing the problem, and
4. monitoring progress.

For readers who desire a more comprehensive description of the tools presented below, please refer to the references and resources at the end of this chapter.

Identifying Customer Expectations

As described in Chapter 2, customer focus is one of the three principles of quality management. Identifying and understanding customer expectations and requirements are essential components of this principle. Asking and observing are the most informal ways to identify patient needs and expectations. Scanning the published literature for information on customer expectations can help a manager avoid reinventing the wheel. For example, the Picker Institute was established in 1987 to promote patient-focused care and to provide information to healthcare organizations about patient-focused approaches. On the basis of information obtained from focus groups, literature, and health professionals, the Picker Institute has identified and defined specific patient requirements, also called dimensions of care (Gerteis et al. 1993a). For the inpatient setting, those dimensions of care are as follows (Gerteis et al. 1993b):

- Respect for patients' values, preferences, and expressed needs
- Coordination and integration of care
- Information, communication, and education
- Physical comfort
- Emotional support and alleviation of fear and anxiety
- Involvement of family and friends
- Transition and continuity

Although the U.S. division of the organization closed in 2001, the dimensions of care described by the Picker Institute still provide an excellent starting point for any healthcare manager to begin a customer-focused improvement effort. Depending on the organization's needs and resources, a deeper understanding of patient requirements may be obtained through focus groups and other qualitative research methods.

Once patient expectations are known, they must be translated into product or service features to ensure that they are being met on a consistent basis for all customers who interface with that product or service. As consumers, many readers are already acquainted with this concept. Internet banking is one example of how financial organizations have created new service features to meet customer expectations for convenient, low-hassle banking services. Experienced healthcare organizations are continually improving their abilities to translate patient expectations into service and product features.

For example, most healthcare providers and employees would describe themselves as "caring"; however, what does caring mean, and how is it expressed by all employees who interact with patients? In one multiphysician practice, caring was defined by the following behaviors: calling patients by name, looking at patients when talking to them, escorting patients to the examination rooms, explaining to patients what they could expect during the visit, and explaining to patients the reasons for any delays experienced during the visit. Office staff (i.e., receptionist, nurses, business office employees, and physicians) were trained and expected to demonstrate these behaviors. In this way, while allowing for individual staff styles and personalities, the practice could ensure that each patient received a consistent level of caring each time he or she visited the office.

Providers of women's specialty care have been particularly effective in translating customer expectations into service features because obstetrics patients have been vocal over the years about their needs and expectations of care providers and facilities. Managers responsible for other clinical areas may gain valuable insights from labor and delivery room design, visiting policies, and prenatal/postpartum education efforts. Labor and delivery processes may help managers better understand the concept of translating patient requirements into actual service features and product design (see Table 3.1).

Documenting a Process

Some of the most valuable improvement tools are those that help managers and teams better understand work processes. It is not uncommon to carry out a process because "that is how we have always done it" or because a certain way of doing things has simply evolved over time. Before a process can be improved, understanding what the current process entails is essential. Using any of the tools described in this section not only provides the opportunity to document the process but also to discuss, question, and clarify perceptions or misconceptions about the process.

A *process* is "a sequence of steps which transform some input into a final output" (Scholtes, Joiner, and Streibel 1996). Benefits of documenting a process include the following:

- Providing a visual picture of the process
- Distinguishing the distinct steps of the process
- Identifying unnecessary steps in the process
- Understanding vulnerabilities—where breakdowns, mistakes, or delays are likely to occur—in a process
- Detecting rework loops that contribute to inefficiency and quality waste

Three tools for documenting processes are described in this section: a process flowchart, a workflow diagram, and lead-time analysis.

Process Flowchart

A *process flowchart* is a picture of the sequence of steps in a process. Different steps are represented by different-shaped symbols. An oval indicates the

Customer Requirement (Picker Dimension of Care)	Service/Product Feature
Involvement of family and friends	Postpartum or labor/delivery/recovery/postpartum room size is large enough to accommodate more than one visitor
	Furniture in patient rooms includes a pullout sofa or cot for father/significant other
	Policies designed for flexible and "safe" visiting hours for grandparents, siblings, and friends (e.g., after screening for infectious illness)
Transition and continuity	Hospital preregistration in advance of admission
	Prenatal and postpartum educational offerings Follow-up nurse phone calls

TABLE 3.1

Translating Customer Requirements Into Service Features (Example: Women's Service)

start and end of the process, a rectangle indicates a process action step, and a diamond indicates a decision that must be made in the process. Depending on the decision, the process follows different paths.

Figure 3.2 illustrates an example of a simple flowchart documenting the process of getting out of bed in the morning. The oval labeled "Start" indicates the beginning of the process. The first step in the process is represented by the rectangle labeled "Alarm goes off." The second step is a decision step represented by the diamond labeled "Too tired?" The steps are connected by arrows that indicate the relationships between the steps. If the answer to the question "Too tired?" is "No," then the next step is "Get out of bed," and the process ends. If the answer to the question "Too tired?" is "Yes," the process follows an alternate path to the step labeled "Hit snooze alarm," which in turn leads back to the first step in the process ("Alarm goes off"). This alternate path is referred to as a rework loop and may be a clue to inefficiencies or unnecessary duplication in the process. Clinicians may already be familiar with this tool, as many clinical algorithms and guidelines are communicated using process flowcharts.

An example of a clinical guideline is shown in Figure 3.3. This particular guideline is one of many developed by the Institute for Clinical Systems Improvement, a nonprofit organization that provides quality

FIGURE 3.2

Simple Process
Flowchart

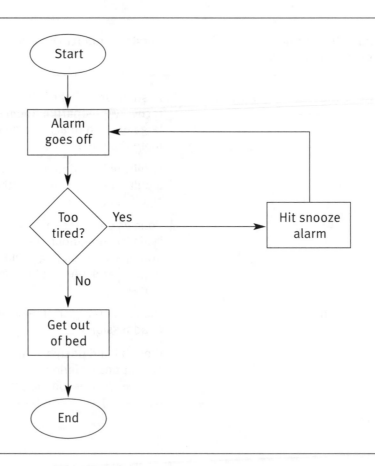

improvement services to medical groups in the state of Minnesota (Institute for Clinical Systems Improvement 2003a; 2003b). The flowchart format displays the sequence of interventions, steps, and decisions that the clinical provider makes in evaluating and treating an acute myocardial infarction.

A deployment flowchart is useful when the steps in a single process are carried out by different people, departments, or organizations. Efforts to improve coordination of process steps may be enhanced by identifying, documenting, and understanding the essential hand-offs that occur in a process. Figure 3.4 illustrates a deployment flowchart for a surgical procedure; in this example, the anesthesiologists wanted to reduce delays between surgical procedures. In a deployment flowchart, the steps in the process are documented with the same symbols used in a process flowchart. The columns in which the symbol is located represent the individual or group responsible for carrying out that step in the process. By using a deployment flowchart, steps occurring in parallel (i.e., those steps above the bold line) can be shown and so can the amount of time the patient spent with each member of the staff in the process, which is represented by the time labels (i.e., Time 1, Time 2) at the bottom of each column. In this way, delays can be readily tracked to their source and, in turn, targeted for improvement.

Workflow Diagram

A *workflow diagram* is a tool used to document how people or things actually move through the physical workspace. This tool is especially useful when it becomes difficult to "see the forest for the trees."

A workflow diagram was instrumental in improving patient flow in an ambulatory surgery unit redesign effort. The unit was an outpatient facility located within a tertiary hospital. The unit location and design had been chosen to be close to a public entrance with automobile access; however, because other patients and staff also used this entrance, many got lost in the ambulatory surgery unit or used the unit as a thoroughfare to other destinations in the hospital. A common comment heard from nurses in the ambulatory surgery unit was "Why does it feel as busy as an emergency department here?"

The nurse manager acquired an official floor plan from the maintenance and engineering department and began mapping the patient flow with simple lines. She found herself drawing long lines from the satellite laboratory that serviced the ambulatory surgery unit and was located at one end of the unit to the outside entrance that was located at the other end of the unit. Upon further investigation, she realized that the non-surgery patient traffic had steadily increased over the years as physicians in the office complex across the street found it convenient to send their own patients to this satellite laboratory for testing. The nurse manager realized that it was this outpatient laboratory traffic that was contributing to the hustle and bustle of activity normally felt only in higher intensity areas such as the emergency department. Once the workflow diagram was completed, the solution became obvious: move the satellite laboratory from the end of the unit that was *furthest* from the outside entrance to the end of unit that was *closest* to the outside entrance.

A workflow diagram also proved useful in the redesign of a laboratory's services. The large laboratory consisted of many smaller specialty laboratories, such as chemistry, cytology, hematology, and bacteriology. Sometimes specimens went to a single area only; however, a specimen was often sent to multiple specialties that each took their portion of the sample and then passed it along to the next area. Early in the redesign process, the team used a workflow diagram to map the flow of specimens within the laboratory facility. The overlapping and backtracking lines drawn on the floor plan became affectionately known to the team as the "plate of spaghetti" (see Figure 3.5). Although the team had sensed that the location of the specialty laboratories in relation to each other was not quite right, the workflow diagram concretely illustrated the inefficiencies and

FIGURE 3.3

Institute for Clinical Systems Improvement Health Care Guideline: Treatment of Acute Myocardial Infarction

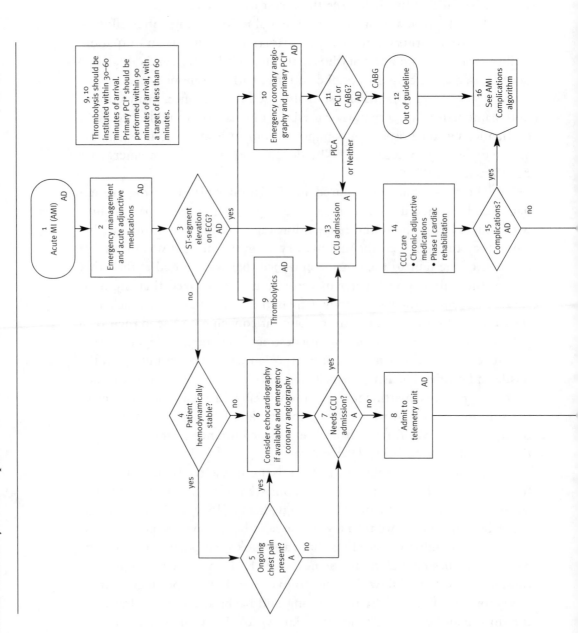

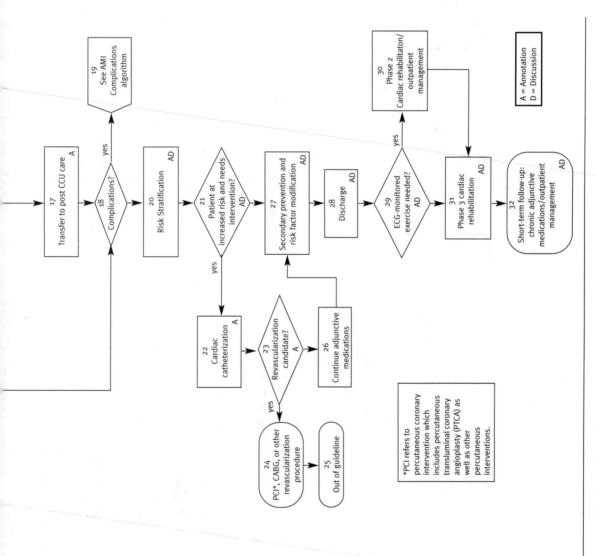

A = Annotation
D = Discussion

17
Transfer to post CCU care
A

18
Complications?

yes

19
See AMI
Complications
algorithm

20
Risk Stratification
AD

21
Patient at
increased risk and needs
intervention?
AD

yes

22
Cardiac
catheterization
A

23
Revascularization
candidate?
A

yes

24
PCI*, CABG, or other
revascularization
procedure

25
Out of guideline

26
Continue adjunctive
medications

27
Secondary prevention and
risk factor modification
AD

28
Discharge
AD

29
ECG-monitored
exercise needed?
AD

yes

30
Phase 2
Cardiac rehabilitaton/
outpatient
management

31
Phase 3 cardiac
rehabilitation
AD

32
Short-term follow-up:
chronic adjunctive
medications/outpatient
management
AD

*PCI refers to
percutaneous coronary
intervention which
includes percutaneous
transluminal coronary
angioplasty (PTCA) as
well as other
percutaneous
interventions.

FIGURE 3.4
Deployment
Flowchart
Example

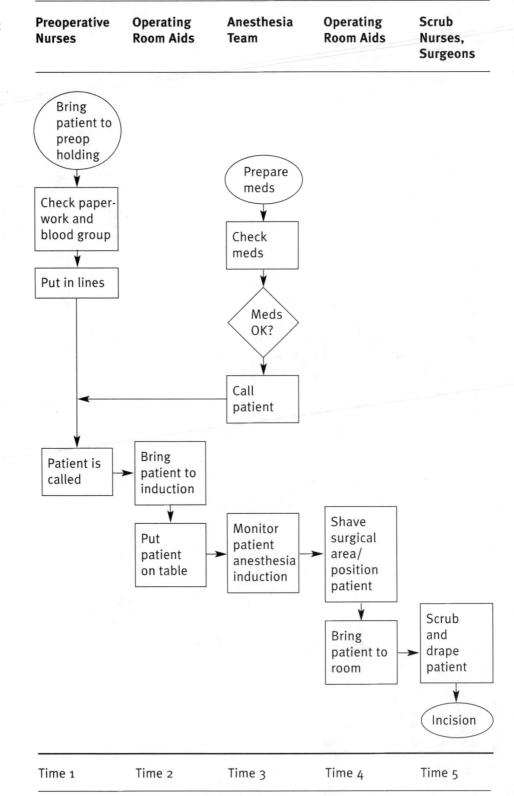

unnecessarily complicated and confusing flow. In turn, ideas about how and where to relocate equipment and people to streamline flow and maximize efficiency became evident to the team members (Kelly 1998).

Lead-Time Analysis

A *lead-time analysis* is a tool used by General Motors' (GM) PICOS quality efforts that has been taught to healthcare workers during collaborative efforts in which PICOS staff assisted hospitals in their improvement efforts (Pougnet 1996). The lead-time analysis tool (see Figure 3.6), like a workflow diagram, is useful in understanding the physical path taken during a process.

The user of this tool physically walks through the process that a document, a specimen, a piece of equipment, or a patient would follow. If a manager is using a lead-time analysis to study the patient admission process, he or she would start at the same place as the patient by driving to the hospital parking garage. In the first column of the lead-time analysis (Step #), the steps of the process are numbered in sequence. In the second column (Process Step Description), the actual action that takes place at this point is described. The first step of the admission process, for example, may be described as "Drive around parking lot until an empty space is found."

The rest of the columns are then completed for the step: the time it takes to complete the step, the distance covered for that step or the distance between steps, the number of times that step occurs (during the process or throughout day), and if the step adds value to the process. (GM defines *value-added* as "something that the customer is willing to pay for" [Pougnet 1996].)

Because in healthcare certain steps of a process may be dictated by a regulatory requirement, this adapted version of GM's lead-time analysis includes a column for regulatory requirement. Although a customer may not be willing to pay for this step of the process, it is essential that it remains. Another addition to the GM version of the tool is to evaluate the process step in relation to the organizational mission, vision, and values. Clearly, the process step described in this patient admission example, where it took 15 minutes and three trips around the parking garage to find a parking place, is not aligned with an organization that tries to be patient focused.

As with the workflow diagram, the actual process of completing the tool, not just reviewing the information written on the form, often leads to identifying obvious areas for improvement. In the laboratory redesign effort described previously, the team also used the lead-time analysis tool. One team member completed it to better understand the journey taken by test results once he had finished his analysis of a specimen. He knew that he completed the analysis in a timely fashion and was baffled by the numerous complaints that his specialty laboratory received about delayed results. The lead-time analysis revealed a cumbersome process that caused a printed

FIGURE 3.5
Workflow
Diagram
Example

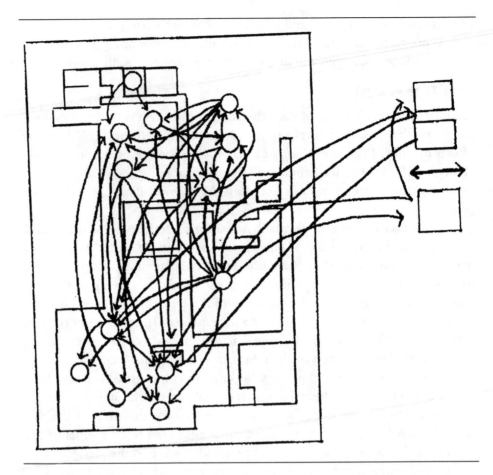

laboratory result to make a three- to five-day journey through the interoffice mail system to the physicians' offices across the street. As he continued to explore the process, this technician found that this was the case for many of the smaller offices served by the laboratory. Although the larger clinics may receive results more quickly, because they had a printer interface with the laboratory's information system, the smaller offices depended on interoffice or postal service mail. When results were not received in a timely manner, an office staff member would usually call the laboratory and someone would have to look up and print the results and then fax the results to the caller. Documenting the process using the lead-time analysis revealed the duplication of work, the quality waste, and the source of delays in physicians and patients receiving their test results. Understanding the process helped the team identify and implement solutions to reduce delays in clinicians' receiving the test results (Kelly 1998).

Diagnosing the Problem

The following tools can help with the documentation, organization, and prioritization of possible causes of a problem: Fishbone diagram, check sheet, and Pareto diagram.

FIGURE 3.6
Lead-Time Analysis Grid

Process/Product Description _____   Page ____ of ____

Step #	Process Step Description	Time	Distance	Quantity	Value-added	Non-Value-added	Regulatory Requirement	Aligned with VVM
1	Drive around parking lot until an empty space is found	15 min.	0.5 mi.	3		✓	No	No

Date completed: _____   Prepared by: _____

Source: Reprinted with permission from General Motors Corporation, Warren, Michigan.

Fishbone Diagram

A *cause-and-effect diagram* is a tool for identifying and organizing the possible causes of a problem in a structured format (Scholtes, Joiner, and Streibel 1996). Because this diagram resembles a fish (the problem represents the head and the causes represent the bones), it is also referred to as a *fishbone diagram*. The problem is written on the far right of the diagram. Categories of causes are represented by the diagonal lines (bones) connected to the horizontal line (spine), which lead to the problem (head). Figures 3.7 and 3.8 illustrate two common ways to draw and label a fishbone diagram (Scholtes, Joiner, and Streibel 1996). Managers may find it useful to label problems related to service processes according to the Four Ps: People, Procedures, Policies, and Plan. Categories labeled with the Four Ms—Manpower, Materials, Methods, and Machinery—may be better suited for problems associated with production processes or technology.

Figure 3.9 illustrates an example of a fishbone diagram used by a multidisciplinary improvement team charged with addressing the problem of inconsistent patient identification prior to rendering clinical services. In this example, the Four Ps were used as the general categories to organize the causes. Detailed causes are identified and represented by the small bones of the fish. Identification band and care issues may be found as a cause under the category labeled "People." When this cause is broken down further, three additional causes are documented: Edema (swelling that may be related to the patient's clinical status), Hidden (covered with sterile drapes in the operating room), and IV line (wristband interfering with site of intravenous line insertion or stabilization).

Check Sheet

Although many organizations have electronic systems from which to obtain data reports, smaller organizations or physician practices may be limited in their ability to collect data in electronic formats. Managers must remember that valuable information may be obtained using tools such as talking to employees and using pencil-and-paper data collection to better understand a problem. A check sheet is one of these "low tech" tools. A check sheet is "a simple data collection form on which you make tally marks to indicate how often something occurs" (Scholtes, Joiner, and Streibel 1996).

Figure 3.10 shows an example of a check sheet used by an obstetrics and gynecology clinic to track different types of phone calls to the clinic. In this case, the clinic manager had been receiving numerous complaints from patients that they were unable to get through when phoning the clinic. Although the phone company could provide aggregate data helpful to evaluate productivity (e.g., number of total calls, average time on hold, number of interrupted calls [caller hanging up while on hold]), this type of information would not help the manager to identify the cause or solve the patients' complaint. The manager's first step was to ask employ-

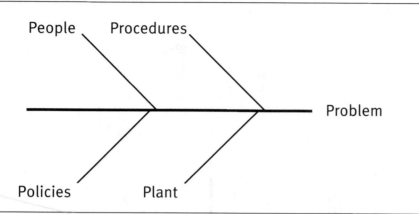

FIGURE 3.7
Fishbone
Diagram: The
Four Ps

ees to identify the types of calls they received in a typical day. The manager then needed to collect data on the frequency of each of these types of calls. When employees are asked to collect data for a short period of time with the intent of addressing a work problem they are concerned with, they will typically consent to the request. The clinic's phone room staff was asked to complete the data-collection check sheet each day for a week.

A user-friendly check sheet should be easy to understand, accessible to the user, and able to be completed quickly.

Pareto Chart

Once data about a problem have been collected, the manager may use a Pareto chart to help prioritize improvement interventions and to focus activities on the highest leverage areas. A *Pareto chart* is a simple bar graph that displays data in descending order from left to right. Figure 3.11 illustrates a Pareto chart for the data collected on the check sheet by the clinic's phone room staff. Graphing the data this way helped the clinic manager to select specific interventions that would best address the problem.

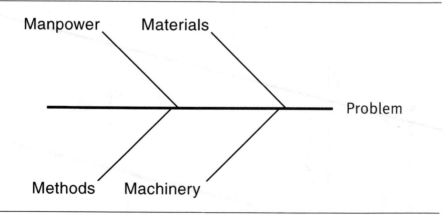

FIGURE 3.8
Fishbone
Diagram:
The Four Ms

FIGURE 3.9
Fishbone Diagram Example

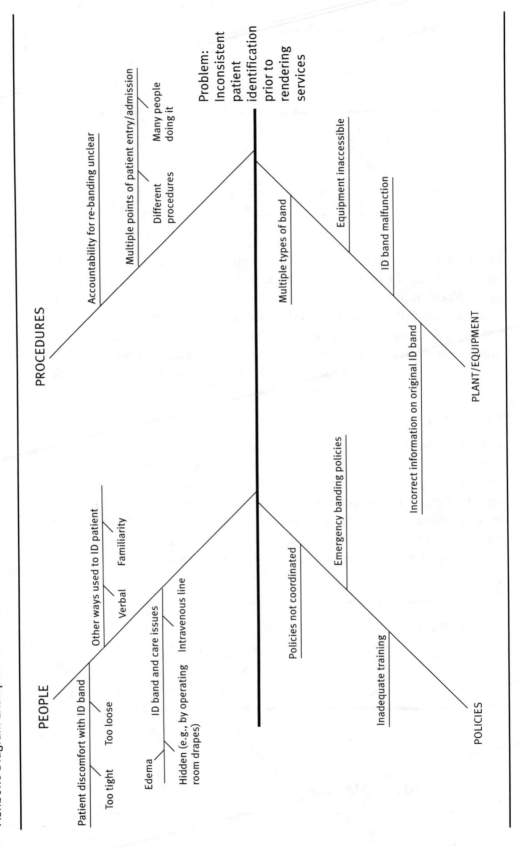

FIGURE 3.10

Check Sheet Example

OB/GYN Phone Room
Data Collection Sheet: Volume of Calls by Type

Name _____   Day of the week: M   T   W   Th   Fr

Type of Call	8:00–9:00 a.m.	9:01–10:00 a.m.	10:01–11:00 a.m.	11:01 a.m.–12:00 p.m.	12:01–1:00 p.m.	1:01–2:00 p.m.	2:01–3:00 p.m.	3:01–4:00 p.m.	4:01–5:00 p.m.
Make an appointment									
Call for nurse: patient									
Call for nurse: nonpatient									
Call for MD: patient									
Call for MD: nonpatient									
Personal call									
Wrong number									
Asking for a phone number									
Other									

Instructions: Please place a tic mark for each phone call you receive in the appropriate time and type box. Use the back of this sheet for comments and/or to describe reasons for "other" calls.

First, the phone team members identified that, although the most frequent number of calls were about making appointments, not all of these calls actually resulted in an actual appointment being scheduled. Because the physicians provided their schedules 30 days in advance, any caller requesting or requiring an appointment beyond this time frame was asked to call back. For a patient to call three times to obtain a single appointment was not uncommon. In addition, the time spent telling patients to call back could have been used for other purposes, thereby increasing the productivity of the phone room staff. Next, the manager was able to identify an unintended consequence of a previous intervention. In an effort to create a more patient-friendly clinic, intercom paging of the nurses and physicians had been eliminated. When the Pareto chart showed that calls for nurses and physicians accounted for about 25 percent of total calls, it helped explain why many patients could not get through in a timely way: the phones were placed on hold for excessive amounts of time while the phone room staff searched for nurses and doctors in this large clinic to notify them of their phone calls.

Readers may wonder why the manager needed a Pareto chart to discover this problem. An important lesson for managers who are beginning improvement efforts is to ensure that improving one problem in one area does not create a problem in a different area. In this case, a new medical director was very distressed by the noise and disruption of the pages. In an effort to satisfy the medical director, the manager did not think to implement an alternative method of communication between the phone staff and the clinical providers.

The second most frequent type of call fell under the category of "Other." For every two calls for an appointment, the phone room was receiving one "other" call, the purpose of which was not readily explained. This realization prompted the manager to further investigate the "other" category to gain insights into the type of calls interfering with appointment-generating calls or calls related to clinical questions. Rather than lobby for more phone room staff, which was the solution proposed initially, the clinic manager set about negotiating with the physicians to receive their schedules further in advance, instituting an internal pager system to replace the overhead intercom, and identifying the reasons for the "other" phone calls.

Monitoring Progress

A *run chart* is a graphic representation of data over time and assists in the monitoring of progress, both after an improvement intervention and ongoing operations. On a run chart, the x-axis represents the time interval (e.g., day, month, quarter, year) and the y-axis represents the variable of interest. Displaying data on a run chart also enables a manager to more readily detect patterns or unusual occurrences in the data.

Figure 3.12 illustrates a run chart of monthly patient visits to a mammography center. The center's staff had been complaining about being very

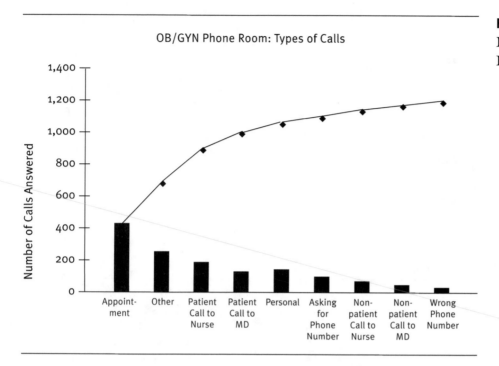

OB/GYN Phone Room: Types of Calls

FIGURE 3.11
Pareto Chart
Example

busy for several months. The manager needed to determine if the increase in visits was here to stay or if it was a passing phenomenon. She converted the volume statistics from a series of monthly management reports to a run chart and was then able to determine the answer to her question. A "once every hundred years" snowstorm had hit the city the previous January and literally shut down business for four days. The center's current busyness was a reflection of the need to reschedule appointments that were cancelled as a result of the snowstorm. The overall volumes for the year were still on track; it was the monthly distribution of visits that had been affected by this unusual and explainable event.

Figure 3.13 illustrates another example of a run chart. In this case, the internal medicine clinic of a large multispecialty physician practice implemented changes in its workflow to reduce patient waiting times and improve patient satisfaction. The run chart shows that patient satisfaction actually decreased the first month after the changes were implemented in September. This is not uncommon because new processes often take time to stabilize as a result of staff learning curves and adjustments. Managers must not overreact to one month's worth of data but should continue to track results over time to see the pattern of performance once the process has stabilized. This run chart demonstrates that although patient satisfaction dropped initially, in subsequent months it stabilized at a higher average level and that more consistent performance became apparent from month to month.

FIGURE 3.12

Run Chart
Example for
Breast
Imaging
Services:
Diagnostic and
Screening
Visits

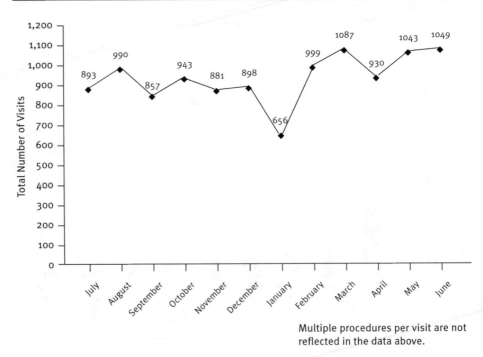

Multiple procedures per visit are not
reflected in the data above.

FIGURE 3.13

Run Chart
Example for
Overall Patient
Satisfaction:
Internal
Medicine
Clinic

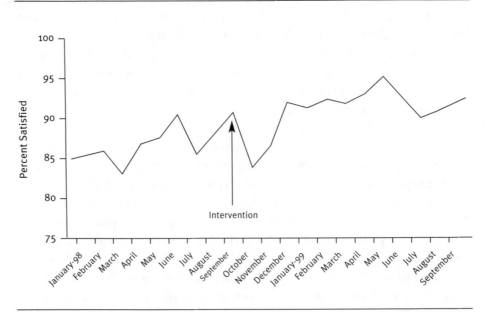

Conclusion

This chapter provides a general overview of common continuous improvement tools. Just as clinical education includes "practice labs" to promote learning while minimizing patient harm, students and practicing managers alike may also learn quality tools and approaches in practice labs before they test these tools in ways that affect their organization; employees; and, ultimately, patients.

The exercise in this chapter may be viewed as such a lab for managers as they practice an improvement process step by step. Section II introduces quality management from a systems approach. Chapter 4 explores concepts of systems thinking and dynamic complexity as expressed in healthcare organizations.

Companion Readings

Gerteis, M., S. Edgman-Levitan, J. D. Walker, D. M. Stoke, P. D. Cleary, and T. L. Delbanco. 1993. "What Patients Really Want." *Health Management Quarterly* 15 (3): 2–6.

Scholtes, P. R., B. L. Joiner, and B. J. Streibel. 1996. *The Team Handbook*, 2nd Edition, Chapter 2 and Appendix A. Madison, WI: Joiner Associates, Inc.

References

Gerteis, M. S., S. Edgman-Levitan, J. D. Walker, D. M. Stoke, P. D. Cleary, and T. L. Delbanco. 1993a. "What Patients Really Want." *Health Management Quarterly* 15 (3): 2–6.

Gerteis, M., S. Edgman-Levitan, J. Daley, and T. L. Delbanco, eds. 1993b. *Through the Patient's Eyes: Understanding and Promoting Patient-Centered Care*. San Francisco: Jossey-Bass.

Institute for Clinical Systems Improvement. 2003a. "About ICSI." [Online information; retrieved 06/28/02]. http://www.icsi.org/about/.

———. 2003b. "Treatment of Acute Myocardial Infarction." [Online information; retrieved 01/31/03]. http://www.icsi.org/knowledge/.

Institute for Healthcare Improvement. 2003. "Breakthrough Series Collaboratives." [Online information; retrieved 06/06/02]. http://www.ihi.org/collaboratives/breakthroughseries/.

Juran, J. M. 1989. *Juran on Leadership for Quality: An Executive Handbook*. New York: The Free Press.

Kelly, D. L. 1998. "Reframing Beliefs About Work and Change Processes in Redesigning Laboratory Services." *Joint Commission Journal on Quality Improvement* 24 (9): 154–67.

Langley, G. J., K. M. Nolan, T. W. Nolan, C. L. Norman, and L. P. Provost. 1996. *The Improvement Guide: A Practical Approach to Enhancing Organizational Performance*. San Francisco: Jossey-Bass.

Pougnet, T. 1996. General Motors workshop given at Intermountain Healthcare, Salt Lake City, Utah, May 20–23.

Scholtes, P. R., B. L. Joiner, and B. J. Streibel. 1996. *The Team Handbook,* 2nd Edition. Madison, WI: Joiner Associates, Inc.

Walton, M. 1986. *The Deming Management Method.* New York: The Putnam Publishing Group.

Exercise

Objective: To practice quality improvement tools by applying them to an improvement effort in an ambulatory care setting

Instructions:

1. Read the following case study.
2. Follow the instructions at the end of the case.

Case Study

Background

You have just been brought in to manage a portfolio of several specialty clinics in a large multiphysician group practice in an academic medical center. The clinics reside in a multiclinic facility that houses primary care and specialty practices as well as a satellite laboratory and radiology and pharmacy services. The practice provides the following centralized services for each of its clinics: registration, payer interface (e.g., authorization), and billing. The CEO of the practice has asked you to initially devote your attention to Clinic X to improve its efficiency and patient satisfaction

Access Process

A primary care physician (or member of the office staff), patient, or family member calls the receptionist at Clinic X to request an appointment. If the receptionist is in the middle of helping a patient in person, the caller is asked to hold. The receptionist then asks the caller, "How may I help you?" If the caller is requesting an appointment within the next month, the appointment date and time is made and given verbally to the caller. If the caller asks additional questions, the receptionist provides answers. The caller is then given the toll-free preregistration phone number and asked to preregister before the date of the scheduled appointment. If the requested appointment is beyond a 30-day period, the caller's name and address are put in a "future file" because physician availability is given only one month in advance. Every month, the receptionist reviews the future file and schedules an appointment for each person on the list, and a confirmation is automatically mailed to the caller.

When a patient preregisters, the financial office is automatically notified and can perform the necessary insurance checks and authorizations for the appropriate insurance plan. If the patient does not preregister, when the patient arrives in the clinic on the day of the appointment and checks in with the specialty clinic receptionist, he or she is asked to first go to the central registration area to register. If there is an obvious problem with authorization, it is corrected before the patient returns to the specialty clinic waiting room.

Receptionist's Point of View

The receptionist has determined that the best way to not inconvenience the caller is to keep him or her on the phone for as short an amount of time as possible. The receptionist also expresses frustration with the fact that there are too many things to do at once.

Physician's Point of View

The physician thinks that too much of his or her time is spent on paperwork and chasing down authorizations. The physician senses that appointments are always running behind and that patients are frustrated, no matter how nice he or she is to them.

Patients' Point of View

Patients are frustrated when asked to wait in a long line to register, which makes them late for their appointment, and when future file appointments are scheduled without their input. As a result of this latter factor, and work or childcare conflicts, patients often just do not show up for these scheduled appointments.

Office Nurse's Point of View

This nurse feels that he or she is playing catch up all day long and explaining delays. The nurse also wishes there was more time for teaching.

Billing Office's Point of View

The office feels that some care is given that is not reimbursed because of inaccurate or incomplete insurance or demographic information or that care is denied authorization after the fact.

Data

On the Picker Institute web site (http://www.pickersymposium.org/care.asp), you find the following patient expectations/dimensions of care for both adults and children in their outpatient experiences with a hospital or clinic outpatient appointment:

*   Access
*   Information and education
*   Respect for patients' values, preferences, and expressed needs
*   Coordination and integration of care
*   Emotional support
*   Continuity and transition

The clinics have just begun to monitor performance data, and you have one quarter's worth of data for the clinic:

Overall satisfaction with visit	82%
Staff is courteous and helpful	90%
Waiting room time is less than 15 minutes	64%
Examination room waiting time is less than 15 minutes	63%
Patient no-show rate	20%
Patient cancellation rate	11%
Provider cancellation rate	10%
Preregistration rate	16%
Average number of patient visits per day	16
Range of patient visits per day	10–23

Instructions

1. Completely read all of the instructions.
2. Decide which problem you want to focus on as your first priority—the goal for your improvement team.
3. Identify the team members that you would want to participate in this effort and what fundamental knowledge they should bring to the process.
4. Document the current process using a process flowchart.
5. Identify your customers and their expectations.
6. Prioritize opportunities to improve by doing the following:
   a. completing a root-cause analysis using a fishbone diagram with the following categories: People (patients), People (staff/employees), Policies and Procedures, and Plant (facilities/equipment);
   b. describing how you would collect data to determine where your greatest opportunity for improvement would be; and
   c. designing a Pareto chart from the data given in the table above (you may also use hypothetical data to design your Pareto chart).
7. Review the following change concepts (Langley et al. 1996) and identify the ones that may apply to your process:
   • Eliminate waste (things that are not used, intermediaries, unnecessary duplication)
   • Improve workflow (minimize handoffs, move steps in the process closer together, find and remove bottlenecks, do tasks in parallel, adjust to high and low volumes)
   • Manage time (reduce set-up time and waiting time)
   • Manage variation (create standard processes where appropriate)
   • Design systems to avoid mistakes (use reminders)
8. Improve the process and document the improved process with a process flowchart or workflow diagram.
9. Decide what you will measure and briefly describe how you would collect the data.

10. You have completed the "Plan" phase of the Shewhart Cycle. Describe briefly how you would complete the rest of the Plan-Do-Check/Study-Act cycle.

11. Save your answers to each part of this exercise. This will become the documentation of your improvement effort.

THE SYSTEMS APPROACH

A SYSTEMS PERSPECTIVE OF QUALITY MANAGEMENT

Objectives

- To introduce the concept of systems thinking
- To introduce the concept of dynamic complexity
- To provide examples that illustrate dynamic complexity in healthcare
- To explore the implications of dynamic complexity for healthcare managers

As individuals accumulate years of experience in the healthcare field, they begin to see the recurring problems—sometimes within an individual organization, sometimes across the entire industry. Problems thought to be solved by one manager may come back at a later time for a different manager. A CEO of a large hospital may eliminate the case management department to meet necessary budget cuts for the year; three years later, the new CEO of the same hospital may create a case management department to address numerous problems with the patient discharge process. Consider the following situation:

> The hospital faces a number of problems concerning the nursing staff . . . one major problem is . . . attracting and retaining a sufficient professional nursing staff, especially non-supervisory nursing staff . . . . [T]he problem lies in the fact that the number of professional nurses being trained in nursing schools is much too low to meet an ever increasing demand for professional nurses by hospitals and other sources. . . . [B]eing understaffed, hospitals often assign to the professional nurse a rather heavy workload that is not seen as normal or reasonable by many nurses . . . . [A]nother important problem . . . involves the composition of the total nursing staff, the question of optimum balance in the proportions of staff members who are registered nurses, practical nurses, and aides. (Georgopoulos and Mann 1962)

Although this situation may appear to address a manager's current challenges with nursing shortages, the above excerpt was taken from the book *The Community General Hospital,* which was published in 1962! During the more than 40 years since that text was written, healthcare organizations seem to have made little headway in issues related to workforce planning and management. Nursing shortages, for example, have appeared and disappeared in waves in the 1960s, 1970s, 1980s, early 1990s, and again in the early years of the twenty-first century.

Why do budget problems and nursing shortages remain nagging issues for healthcare managers? The reasons lie in the complex nature of healthcare, healthcare organizations, and the healthcare industry. By "complex" we mean the presence of a large number of variables that interact with each other in innumerable ways. In addition to the presence of many variables, healthcare and healthcare systems are characterized by situations in which "cause and effect are not close in time and space and obvious interventions do not produce expected outcomes" (Senge 1990). This characteristic represents another type of complexity, known as *dynamic complexity*. Although an intervention may appear to be the obvious solution at the time, if it does not alter the fundamental behavior of the system that is causing the problem, the solutions are only temporary. As seen in the nursing shortage example, although interventions may offer temporary relief, the problems resurface again and again.

In healthcare, as in other industries, "systems thinking is needed more than ever because we are being overwhelmed with complexity" (Senge 1990). This chapter introduces a systems perspective of quality management that is based on the concepts of systems thinking and dynamic complexity.

Systems Thinking

In Chapter 1, a variety of perspectives surrounding the term "quality" were discussed. Likewise, the term "system" brings with it numerous connotations and perceptions. Depending on the source, system may be defined in a variety of ways in healthcare organizations or in healthcare. In this book, *system* refers to a collection of parts that interact with each other to form an interdependent whole (Kauffman 1980; Scott 1998).

Although a system reflects the whole, "systems thinking is a discipline for *seeing* wholes. It is a framework for seeing interrelationships, rather than things, for seeing patterns of change rather that static 'snapshots'" (Senge 1990). *Systems thinking* acknowledges the large number of parts in a system and the infinite number of ways in which the parts interact as well as the nature of the interactions. Systems thinking implies reading between the elements of a system to understand how they are connected.

Dynamic Complexity

Several system characteristics contribute to the presence of dynamic complexity (Sterman 2000). Five characteristics, predominant in healthcare and healthcare organizations, are described in this section: change, tradeoffs, history dependency, tight coupling, and nonlinearity.

Change

Systems are dynamic—that is, changing. Change occurs at different rates and scales within and among systems, especially in healthcare. Consider three levels of dynamic complexity in healthcare. First, the human system/human body changes continuously. This means that key inputs (patients with a clinical problem) to and the outputs (patients' status after clinical intervention) of our healthcare systems represent moving targets. Second, the organizational contexts in which healthcare and healthcare delivery are carried out are dynamic in nature. Employees move in and out of organizations, research provides an ongoing stream of new clinical interventions, and technological advances offer new clinical and management approaches. Third, the communities and political environments in which we live and in which healthcare organizations operate change—that is, the environment changes with economic cycles, political ideologies, and election cycles.

Implications for Healthcare Managers

From the day a person is born to the day he or she dies, that person is in a constant state of change, growing and developing physiologically and emotionally. No two human systems are exactly alike or precisely predictable in their response to a medical intervention. As a result, functions that may seem straightforward in other industries, such as product standardization, become more difficult for healthcare managers. For example, many organizations use the practice of pharmacy benefits management (PBM, a hospital formulary using a standardized list of drug names and brands to reduce medication expenses). However, when the dynamic nature of patient physiology is introduced, the manager recognizes that in addition to the question, "What are the set of drug names and brands that will be most cost-effective?" he or she also needs to ask, "How should the approved drugs be selected, and what are the consequences to patients?"

To aid in grasping the subtle but important nuances involved in individualizing treatment plans, the metaphor of trying on a pair of blue jeans may be used. People have their own favorite brand of blue jeans that "fit," even though another brand may be advertised as a similar size and style. Likewise, owing to individual personal chemistries, certain medications may work better for one person than for others with similar biochemical structures. The PBM essentially dictates to doctors that the patient may buy only slim-cut size 10 jeans and not relaxed-fit size 10 jeans (Kelly and Pestotnik 1998).

An alternative approach to PBM that takes into account the dynamic nature of patient physiology as well as the need to reduce costs is seen in the computer-assisted management program for antibiotics and other anti-infective agents. With this tool, the computer gathers the extensive and complex information about the patient (e.g., vital signs, laboratory and other diagnostic information) and the medication (e.g., dose, frequency, route, contraindications), the clinical evidence (e.g., relevant published studies, use in other similar patients), and the costs of optional therapies. The software program continually updates the most current version of all the necessary decision elements (patient, medical evidence, costs, and safety considerations) and presents the information to care providers at the point of service so that they may make timely decisions about the most appropriate, safe, and cost-effective intervention (Evans et al. 1998; Mullett et al. 2001).

Trade-Offs

The need to understand the nature of trade-offs may seem unnecessary for managers taught to weigh pros versus cons or opportunities versus risks as they consider organizational decision options. Trade-offs may be seen as an accepted attribute of management. However, an understanding of dynamic complexity can shed light on the system consequences of local management trade-off decisions. Trade-offs are seen in dynamically complex systems because "time delays in feedback channels mean the long-run response of a system to an intervention is often different from its short-run response. High leverage policies often cause worse-before-better behavior, while low leverage policies often generate transitory improvement before the problem grows worse" (Sterman 2000).

Implications for Healthcare Managers

A classic example of a low-leverage policy, as defined above, was published in the *New England Journal of Medicine* (Fitzgerald, Moore, and Dittus 1988). Although a 1988 publication may be viewed as dated, the lessons for managers in this article are even more relevant today than when the study was published.

The advent of prospective payment systems in 1983 drove many hospitals to reduce costs by decreasing their patient length of stay. This article examined the impact of these practices on quality of care for elderly patients with hip fractures. As Table 4.1 summarizes, the variables studied included length of stay, number of physical therapy sessions, functional status measured by the distance in feet that patients could walk, percentage of patients discharged to nursing homes, and percentage of patients still in nursing homes one year after discharge. If a manager in this case defined the healthcare system as "the orthopedic department/unit" or the hospital administrator defined the healthcare system as "this hospital," the intervention chosen to reduce healthcare system costs appeared to be appropriate. In this article, the decision and subsequent interventions to reduce length of stay appeared to be successful; mean hospital stay declined from 21.9 to 12.6 days. In addition, "neither in-hospital mortality nor one-year mortality changed significantly" (Fitzgerald, Moore, and Dittus 1988). Based on these criteria—length of hospital stay, hospital mortality, and one-year mortality—the manager may be confident of a successful cost-reduction strategy.

	Before	After
Length of stay	21.9 days	12.6 days
Physical therapy sessions	7.6	6.3
Functional status (measured by distance in feet walked)	93	38
Percentage of patients discharged to nursing homes	38%	60%
Percentage of patients still in nursing homes one year after discharge	9%	33%

TABLE 4.1

Impact of Low-Leverage Policy: Reducing Hospital Costs by Reducing Hospital Length of Stay

Source: Adapted with permission from Table 2 in "The Care of Elderly Patients With Hip Fracture. Changes Since Implementation of the Prospective Payment System" by J. F. Fitzgerald, P. S. Moore, and R. S. Dittus, in the *New England Journal of Medicine* 319 (21): 1394. Copyright © 1988 Massachusetts Medical Society. All rights reserved.

However, if one defines the healthcare system as including not only the acute phase of care (i.e., orthopedic unit, hospital) but also the downstream providers (i.e., rehabilitation and long-term care) and takes into account how the relationships among all providers influence patient outcomes, the longer-term behavior of the system can be observed. The short-term intervention of reducing length of stay, and in turn reducing physical therapy sessions and functional status, also led to an increase in patients discharged from the hospital directly to nursing homes. The authors concluded that the result was a shift in "much of the rehabilitation burden to nursing homes" (Fitzgerald, Moore, and Dittus 1988) and observed the subsequent increase in the percentage of patients remaining in nursing homes at one year after hospital discharge. Overall costs related to the consumption of healthcare resources for the care of these patients actually increased.

To this finding, the manager may respond, "But my responsibility is only my unit/hospital." From a systems perspective, the acute care manager's responsibility is not simply to the acute care unit or hospital but also for the impact those local decisions have on the rest of the system of which the manager's component is a part. This does not mean that the manager of the orthopedic department or the hospital administrator should not strive to reduce hospital costs. It does mean, however, that managers, financial officers, chief executive officers, and policymakers should be aware of how decisions made and implemented within their domain of responsibility affect other parts of the healthcare system, both positively and negatively. When a negative impact to another part of the system is anticipated, the manager should be proactive in the short term to assist in minimizing the negative effects and to preserve positive patient outcomes. In the case presented in this article, a proactive intervention may have been to ensure that nursing homes had adequate rehabilitation capacity before reducing hospital length of stay.

Other common trade-off challenges for healthcare managers surround the differences between expense and investment decisions within organizations and departments. The long-term effect of a manager's short-term decision may not be felt by another component in the system (e.g., nursing home, patient) as in the previous example but will surface at a certain point in the future within the manager's own department or organization. For example, does the manager sacrifice capital improvements to fund traveling nurses in the short term? Do managers reduce staff education dollars to reduce current expenses? Although choosing traveling nurses and reducing staff development activities may meet the short-term need to reduce expense, these efforts fall into the category of low-leverage policies because the problems of facility aging, staff shortages, and the need for a competent workforce will surely be faced by the manager at a certain point in the future. Without an appreciation of system consequences, one manager may be rewarded for the short-term "success" with a promotion, while his successor inherits the longer-term problem.

In the PBM example, the organization may be willing to trade off the rare adverse medication event for dollar savings realized from product standardization. However, this type of micro (patient level)/macro (organizational level) trade-off that allows for patient status to be potentially compromised may unintentionally contribute to polarization and conflict between clinicians and managers.

History Dependency

Systems are history dependent. In other words, what has happened in the past influences what is occurring in the present. Some actions are reversible, but many actions are not.

Implications for Healthcare Managers

Once again, this characteristic may be seen in both the patient and the organization. For example, even though a person stopped smoking at the age of 40, the effects of 25 years of a two-pack-per-day habit dictate this person's health and care requirements for the rest of his or her life. Individual patient histories influence how a manager interprets performance data. Adjusting clinical outcomes for patient acuity (e.g., presence of comorbidities) or adjusting overall organizational acuity takes into account the patient as a dynamic system and is an essential system tool for data analysis in healthcare (Iezzoni 1997).

Another example of this characteristic is illustrated by how a healthcare organization's past decision to pursue or not pursue electronic information systems affects its ability to meet current information demands and reporting requirements. The ability of the healthcare industry to manage information and report performance pales in comparison to other industries such as financial services. Consider the following perspective:

> If you go to the doctor, the doctor is recording your visit in vegetable pigment on crushed wood fibers. This is literally a medieval method of data storage and retrieval. I ask you, how would you react if you went to a bank and asked for money and someone opened up a big, old ledger and blew it off and said, "Oh, let's see, how much do you have?" (Smith 2002)

The manager must realize not only how past events have shaped current events but also how past decision-making strategies and directions may influence his or her ability to successfully achieve current and future goals. Using the information systems example, if the organization has historically rewarded managers for quarterly or annual financial performance, a large capital investment today for a future financial gain may be very difficult to sell given the reward and decision-making history of the organization.

Tight Coupling

A system is characterized as tightly coupled when "the parts exhibit relatively time-dependent, invariant, and inflexible connections with little slack" (Scott 1998) and "the actors in the system interact strongly with one another" (Sterman 2000).

Implications for Healthcare Managers

Depending on their work histories and backgrounds, students and managers may or may not have experienced a work setting that is tightly coupled. Typically, knowledge work is not considered tightly coupled, while certain production and mechanical processes are considered as such. Although healthcare delivery is typically thought of as a service, many work processes within such an organization are actually closer in nature to production processes than service processes, causing the organization to potentially be considered tightly coupled. Healthcare managers who have never actually worked in a tightly coupled system or environment must learn about and gain an appreciation for this system characteristic to be effective in their roles.

A "code" for a cardiac arrest is an example of a healthcare process that is very tightly coupled. Each person on the team carries out his or her respective steps in this emergency process in a specific order, with many steps dependent on a previous step. An intravenous line must be in place before certain medications can be administered. The patient's age and weight determine the exact dosage of medication to be given; inaccurate calculations can have disastrous results.

Specific work settings and environments in a hospital are also considered tightly coupled, including processes, procedures, and staff in operating rooms and intensive care units. Even the concept of continuum of care implies a certain degree of coupling among the patient, the primary care physician, acute care, long-term care, and home care.

Seemingly benign processes, when viewed from one point of view (that is, in terms of cost or acuity), may actually be considered tightly coupled when viewed another way (that is, in terms of the number of interactions within the system required to successfully and safely complete the process). Studies by the Healthcare Advisory Board have shown that a typical x-ray procedure may take up to 40 steps, involve 15 to 20 employees, and require up to 148 minutes from start to finish (The Advisory Board Company 1992). This example alone begs healthcare managers to include work simplification and job design—techniques that have been used in other industries for years—in all improvement efforts (Hackman and Oldham 1980).

Organizations in industries outside of healthcare that are most commonly identified as tightly coupled include nuclear power plants and aircraft carriers. These work environments pose unique organizational and management challenges. As the study of human error and human factors is becoming more visible and accepted within healthcare practice, managers may increasingly take lessons from what are referred to as high-reliability organizations and bring those lessons back to healthcare settings (Reason 1990, 1997; Roberts 1990; Weick and Sutcliffe 2001).

Nonlinearity

The term *nonlinear* as it refers to a system characteristic means that the "effect is rarely proportional to the cause" (Sterman 2000) and that, because the parts in the system may interact in numerous ways, these interactions may follow "unexpected sequences that are not visible or not immediately comprehensible (Scott 1998).

Implications for Healthcare Managers

A nurse just starting the afternoon shift was the object of an outburst of anger from a patient's family. The nurse related the encounter to a colleague at the nurse's station. "All I did was say, 'Hello!'" This situation may bring to mind the old cliché "the straw that broke the camel's back." In fact, this cliché is an accurate description of the encounter.

The patient and her family had accumulated a sequence of unsatisfactory experiences during the hospital stay, so all it took was one more encounter to trigger their anger. The afternoon nurse, although this was the first time he had met the family, was the last in a series of interactions between the patient and the healthcare system that caused this family to use the nurse as a target of their frustration. Now, if the patient complains to the manager about this nurse, what can the manager do? If the manager does not have an appreciation for the nonlinear nature of systems, he or she may be tempted to discipline the nurse. However, if the manager does have an appreciation for the nonlinear nature of systems, he or she may try to recreate with the family the sequence of events that, although each was relatively harmless when considered individually, when linked together with the family's situation contributed to an extremely dissatisfying experience. From this investigation, the manager may identify areas that can be improved to enhance the patient's overall experience with the care delivery process.

Another example of the nonlinear nature of systems may be seen in strategies used to reduce personnel expense in healthcare organizations. Because personnel expenses comprise such a large percentage of operating budgets, changing the "staff mix"—that is, reducing the number of professional staff (i.e., registered nurses, medical technologists, pharmacists) and increasing the proportion of assistive personnel (i.e., nurses' aides, laboratory assistants, pharmacy technicians)—is a common cost-cutting intervention. When this intervention is studied from a systems perspective, however, the resulting sequences of activities and their interrelationships are more readily seen. The unplanned consequences of this cost-cutting strategy in one organization included an increase in the overall employee turnover rate because of the high turnover among the entry-level, assistive personnel group. Because this cost-cutting strategy was used by managers across different types of professions and departments, the stress and cost of continuously recruiting, hiring, and training new employees more than offset the savings hoped for from lowering the average hourly wage. When viewed from one department's point of view, the cost-reduction strategy may appear to be reasonable; however, when the compounding effect of this cost-cutting strategy is viewed across the entire organization, the strategy designed to reduce costs is actually undermining the organization's ability to do so (Kelly 1999).

The nonlinear characteristics of the larger healthcare system can be seen when other consequences of this particular cost-cutting strategy are examined:

> . . . because some local schools decide their enrollments based on the current number of job openings in a particular field, hospital staffing decisions made today can affect the number of qualified job applicants available in four to five years. For example, from 1994 to 1996, local hospitals aggressively reduced positions for registered nurses. Applications for enrollment at a local nursing school dropped by 41 percent during the same time period. (Kelly 1999)

This effect was not only seen with nurses but with medical technologists and radiology technicians as well. This realization, gained through a systems perspective of the organization's cost-cutting strategies, prompted the organization to reevaluate its staffing practices and succession planning and to begin aggressively coordinating with local schools to proactively prepare for future staff shortages. This organization began addressing staff shortages a full three years before the staff shortages in healthcare resurfaced as a widespread concern in 2001 (Kelly 1999; Knox, Irving, and Gharrity 2001).

Conclusion

This chapter introduces the concepts of systems thinking and dynamic complexity as they apply to healthcare and healthcare organizations. Chapter 5 expands on the concept of systems thinking by introducing several systems models that managers may use to better understand the relationships among variables within their own organizations. Understanding these system relationships provides insight into the subtle, but powerful, factors that contribute to the organization's ability to progress along the quality continuum. The exercise at the end of this chapter provides readers an opportunity to practice identifying dynamic complexity in a patient care experience.

Companion Readings

Senge, P. M. 1990. "The Leader's New Work: Building Learning Organizations." *Sloan Management Review* (Fall): 149–65.
Weick, K. E., and K. M. Sutcliffe. 2001. *Managing the Unexpected: Assuring High Performance in an Age of Complexity*, 1–23. San Francisco: Jossey-Bass.

References

The Advisory Board Company. 1992. *Re-Engineering the Hospital: CEO Primer on Bottlenecks, Excess Cost and Lost Revenue*. Washington, DC: The Advisory Board Company.
Evans, R. S., S. L. Pestotnik, D. C. Classen, T. P. Clemmer, L. K. Weaver, J. F. Orme, J. F. Lloyd, and J. P. Burke. 1998. "A Computer-Assisted Management Program for Antibiotics and Other Antiinfective Agents." *New England Journal of Medicine* 338 (4): 232–38.
Fitzgerald, J. F., P. S. Moore, and R. S. Dittus. 1988. "The Care of Elderly Patients with Hip Fracture. Changes Since Implementation of the Prospective Payment System." *New England Journal of Medicine* 319 (21): 1392–97.
Georgopoulos, B. S., and F. C. Mann. 1962. *The Community General Hospital*. New York: The MacMillan Company.
Hackman, J. R., and G. R. Oldham. 1980. *Work Redesign*. Reading, MA: Addison-Wesley Publishing Company.

Iezzoni, L. I., ed. 1997. *Risk Adjustment for Measuring Healthcare Outcomes,* 2nd Edition. Chicago: Health Administration Press.

Kauffman, D. R. 1980. *Systems One: An Introduction to Systems Thinking.* Minneapolis, MN: Future Systems, Inc.

Kelly, D. L. 1999. "Systems Thinking: A Tool for Organizational Diagnosis in Healthcare." In *Making It Happen: Stories from Inside the New Workplace,* compiled from *The Systems Thinker Newsletter,* 89–97. Waltham, MA: Pegasus Communications, Inc.

Kelly, D. L., and S. L. Pestotnik. 1998. "Using Causal Loop Diagrams to Facilitate Double Loop Learning in the Healthcare Delivery Setting." Unpublished manuscript.

Knox, S., J. A. Irving, and J. Gharrity. 2001. "The Nursing Shortage—It's Back!" *JONAS Healthcare, Law, Ethics and Regulation* 4 (2): 31.

Mullett, C. J., R. S. Evans, J. C. Christensen, and J. M. Dean. 2001. "Development and Impact of a Computerized Antiinfective Decision Support Program." *Pediatrics* 108 (4): e75.

Reason, J. 1997. *Managing the Risks of Organizational Accidents.* Burlington, VT: Ashgate Publishing Limited.

———. 1990. *Human Error.* Cambridge, MA: Cambridge University Press.

Roberts, K. 1990. "Some Characteristics of One Type of High Reliability Organization." *Organizational Science* 1: 160–76.

Scott, W. R. 1998. *Organizations: Rational, Natural and Open Systems,* 4th Edition. Upper Saddle River, NJ: Prentice Hall.

Senge, P. M. 1990. *The Fifth Discipline: The Art and Practice of the Learning Organization.* New York: Doubleday Currency.

Smith, M. 2002. "Quality Measurement in Healthcare: The Role of Public Reporting." University of North Carolina at Chapel Hill School of Public Health Program on Health Outcomes, 2002 Spring Seminar Series, March 27.

Sterman, J. D. 2000. *Business Dynamics: Systems Thinking and Modeling for a Complex World.* Boston: Irwin McGraw-Hill.

Weick, K. E., and K. M. Sutcliffe. 2001. *Managing the Unexpected: Assuring High Performance in an Age of Complexity.* San Francisco: Jossey-Bass.

Exercise

Objective: To practice identifying dynamic complexity in a patient care experience.

Instructions:

1. Read the case.
2. Review the system characteristics that contribute to dynamic complexity:
    *   Change
    *   Trade-offs
    *   History dependency
    *   Tight coupling
    *   Nonlinearity
3. Explain how these system characteristics are expressed in the case.

Case Study

This case is adapted from Kelly, D. L., and S. L. Pestotnik. 1998. "Using Causal Loop Diagrams to Facilitate Double Loop Learning in the Healthcare Delivery Setting." Unpublished manuscript.

Mrs. B. was a 66-year-old widow living on a fixed income. She had been diagnosed with high blood pressure and osteoporosis. Her private doctor knew her well. When he selected the medication with which to treat her high blood pressure, he took into account her age, the fact that she had osteoporosis, and other issues. He chose a drug that had proven beneficial for patients like Mrs. B. and that had minimum side effects. Mrs. B. did well on the medication for ten years. Her insurance covered the cost of her medication, except for a small out-of-pocket copayment.

The last time Mrs. B. went to her local pharmacy to refill her prescription, she was informed by her pharmacist that her insurance company had contracted with a pharmacy benefits management (PBM) company. (The role of the PBM is to perform a variety of cost-cutting services for health-insurance plans. One of these services is to decide which drugs an insurance company will pay for; the PBM preferred-product list is known as a *formulary.*) Now if Mrs. B. wanted to continue to take the same medication, it would cost her five times her usual copayment. She was quite disturbed because she could not afford this price increase and did not fully understand her insurance company's new policy. The pharmacist offered to call Mrs. B.'s doctor, explain the situation, and ask him whether he would change her prescription to the PBM-preferred brand. When the physician was contacted, he was not aware of the PBM's action and was not completely familiar with the preferred product. The pharmacist discussed Mrs. B.'s predicament with the physician and described the financial consequences of her continuing to receive her original prescription. After this discussion with the pharmacist, the physician concluded that his only option was to approve the switch, which he did.

Mrs. B. began taking the new brand of high blood pressure medicine. One week after starting on the new drug, she developed a persistent cough that aggravated her osteoporosis and caused her rib pain. When the cough and pain continued for another week, Mrs. B. began to take over-the-counter medicines for the pain. She unknowingly opened herself to having a reaction between her blood pressure medication and the pain medication: orthostatic hypertension (lightheadedness when rising from a laying to upright position). One morning on her way to the bathroom, she fainted, fell, and broke her hip. She was admitted to the hospital for surgery, where she developed a urinary tract infection. The infection spread to her repaired hip, which resulted in a bloodstream infection that eventually led to her death.

SYSTEMS MODELS FOR HEALTHCARE MANAGERS

Objectives

- To describe four systems models for healthcare managers
- To discuss selected lessons for healthcare managers from each model

Just as a roadmap provides a picture of how places are connected in a geographic area, systems models can provide a picture for managers of how elements may be connected within an organization. Numerous models provide healthcare managers with a picture of the organizational system in which they work. Different models may resonate with different managers depending on their work settings, backgrounds, and individual preferences. The model that the manager selects is less important than how he or she uses it to begin recognizing, understanding, and anticipating how the parts of the systems interact as a whole.

Four models are presented in this chapter: the Organizational Systems Design model, the Three Core Process model, the Socioecological Framework, and the Baldrige National Quality Program Healthcare Criteria for Performance Excellence.

Organizational Systems Design Model

The most basic system may be characterized by three elements: input(s), a conversion process, and output(s). These elements are demonstrated visually in the simple diagram below:

Input(s) ➡ Conversion process ➡ Output(s)

The Organizational Systems Design (OSD) model, shown in Figure 5.1, illustrates these three essential elements (Axtell and Eckholdt 1992).

The boxes on the left of the figure represent inputs and are labeled as environmental factors and principles of leadership. Environmental factors in healthcare include the characteristics of the community in which an organization operates, market and competitive forces, and regulatory requirements. In OSD, the essential and influential role of leadership is represented as an input to the system and indicated by the label "Principles of the leadership." The ovals on the right of the figure represent outputs and include business outcomes, and behaviors and feelings. These behaviors and feel-ings may refer to those of customers (e.g., customer satisfaction, loyalty), employees (e.g., employee morale, motivation), or other partners (e.g., a desire for ongoing collaboration). The large rectangle in the middle of the figure represent the conversion process. The organization's mission, guid-ing principles, customer focus strategy, and goals and objectives (top por-tion of the rectangle) collectively provide a foundation to guide how the work system is designed. The interconnected boxes (lower portion of the rectangle) represent the components of the work system—that is, how the organization operates to produce products or deliver services. These boxes represent the operating subsystems and their relationships to one another.

The technical subsystem is the technology used to produce the prod-uct or service. In healthcare, the technical subsystem may include tech-nology in the form of equipment (e.g., radiology machines, laboratory ana-lyzers, computers). However, the technical subsystem may also include management technology as it relates to how processes and jobs are designed. The term "structural subsystem" refers to the way people are organized and to the respective policies and procedures defining people's roles and relationships to each other. The information subsystem involves how infor-mation is collected, communicated, reported, and used within the organ-ization. This subsystem may address organizational performance, infor-mation related to patients' clinical status, or the content and manner of management's communication to employees. The people subsystem includes all human resources functions within the organization, such as recruitment, hiring, training, and performance evaluation. The rewards subsystem not only addresses financial compensation but also nonfinancial rewards such as recognition, accomplishment, and respect. The renewal system refers to the organization's process for maintaining and improving its work system over time. All of these subsystems are connected to produce the outputs.

Lessons for Healthcare Managers

The OSD model offers two key lessons to managers. The first lesson is that managers must realize that the elements that make up the center of the model and that enable the conversion of inputs to outputs are labeled as "choices." The term *choice* implies that a particular alternative has been selected from a variety of options. The OSD model provides managers with a framework to better understand organizational choices.

Choices may be conscious or not, supporting an old saying heard around election time: "Not to vote is to vote." Similarly, an organization's mission, guiding principles, customer focus strategy, goals and objectives, and work systems may be consciously designed, may evolve from habit, or may exist by default. If the manager is not pleased with the organization's current outputs, new choices about the elements in this center box of the model can be made. For example, using the OSD model, a manager may be prompted to ask the following questions:

FIGURE 5.1
Organizational
Systems
Design Model

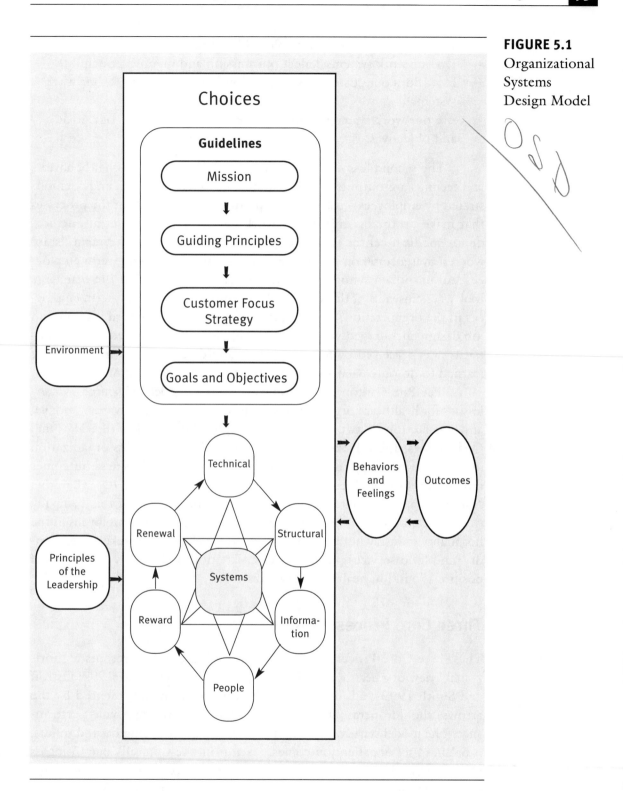

- What are the guiding principles of our organization?
- Do our work systems reflect our mission and guiding principles?
- How does our customer strategy drive choices related to our work systems?
- Are our work systems designed to enable us to achieve our goals and objectives?

The second lesson is that managers must understand that behaviors and feelings are outputs of the system. The behaviors or feelings demonstrated by employees, customers, or partners are the result of the processes that make up the organization's work system. For example, in one academic medical center affiliated with a state university, the term "state worker" was a common descriptor used by managers for long-term employees. An unspoken synonym for state worker was "lazy." If the managers took a systems view of the apparent lack of motivation of long-term employees in the organization, they might have seen that the reward systems and job design encouraged workers to do only what was required. Worker initiative was perceived by managers as insubordination, so workers quickly learned to do only what they were told to do and nothing more.

The Ritz-Carlton Hotel Company is a role model and source of many lessons for healthcare organizations regarding employee motivation, morale, and satisfaction. A two-time winner of the Malcolm Baldrige National Quality Award, the Ritz-Carlton has been able to design its organization in ways that not only result in excellent customer and business outcomes but also result in high employee motivation, pride, and initiative (Baldrige National Quality Program 2001). The accomplishments of this company warrant attention from healthcare managers because most employees in the hospitality industry hold relatively low-paying clerical, housekeeping, laundry, and food services positions, which are not unlike many support staff positions found in healthcare organizations.

Three Core Process Model

The Three Core Process model shown in Figure 5.2 represents a "horizontal" view of a healthcare delivery organization (Kelly et al. 1997; Ostroff and Smith 1992); all processes in the organization (represented by the arrows) should operate in an aligned fashion toward improving performance. The model starts on the right of the figure by defining desired results. A balanced set of patient outcomes, taken from the Clinical Value Compass (Nelson et al. 1996), is used to describe the desired results in clinical outcomes, functional status, satisfaction against need, and cost. Based on lessons from the OSD model, the Three Core Process model also describes organizational culture and behaviors as outcomes or outputs of the organization's work processes.

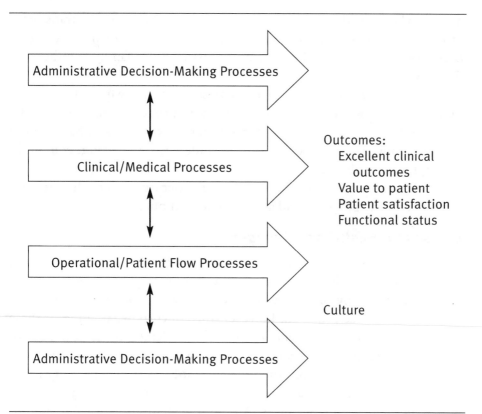

FIGURE 5.2
Three Core
Process Model

According to the Three Core Process model, although many processes take place in a healthcare delivery organization, they may be grouped into three core categories: (1) clinical processes, (2) operational or patient flow processes, and (3) administrative processes.

Clinical/medical processes are the fundamental reasons that patients seek the services of a healthcare organization—that is, to address some clinical need that may include processes related to diagnosis, treatment, prevention, and palliative care. Clinical/medical processes include those under the domain of physicians as well as those under the domain of nonphysicians. This process may be a medical (e.g., physician) process, such as surgery; may be related to improving the individual's functional status, such as physical therapy; may be related to daily care that the individual or family is unable to carry out without help, such as nursing care after an accident; or may be related to receiving special medication or respiratory treatments, such as oxygen and intravenous medication for an individual with pneumonia.

Operational/patient flow processes are those that enable the patient to access the clinical processes during his or her visit or course of stay. This core category includes processes that involve the following: registering and admitting the patient to the facility, administering diagnostic tests, determining what unit the patient goes to and when the patient is transferred or discharged, ensuring that the patient receives meals or medications at the appropriate time, and preparing the patient and family members for discharge.

Administrative decision-making processes occupy two positions in the figure, above and below the other two core processes. In this way, the model illustrates the influence that administrative processes have on the overall organization. These processes include decision making, communication, resource allocation, and performance evaluation.

The arrows linking the three core processes reflect the interdependence of the processes in leading to desired outcomes.

Lessons for Healthcare Managers

The Three Core Process model teaches managers several lessons. First, the interdependent relationships between the three core processes suggest that improvement in any one of these processes has the potential to increase value of the service provided; however, the concurrent targeting of these core processes provides a synergy that can accelerate the achievement of improved outcomes. For example, in one ambulatory surgery unit, the patient length of stay—from the time the patient left the operating room to the time the patient was discharged—was found to be longer than in similar ambulatory surgery units. An improvement effort was initiated to address the postoperative process of care so that the discharge process could be improved and, in turn, the length of stay could be reduced. As the improvement team realized, if patients were being heavily sedated in the operating room and were slow to wake up as a result, then the gains in length of stay could not be fully realized. Likewise, if the physicians implemented a new clinical protocol for anesthesia and pain management but patients still had to wait for the nurses to discharge them, then gains in length of stay again could not be fully realized. Recognizing the interdependence of these two processes and targeting both the discharge process and the anesthesia protocol for improvement allowed the benefits of both improvement efforts to be achieved. Importantly, if the administrative processes did not permit employees to be scheduled away from work to be able to be involved in the quality efforts, neither of the improvements could take place at all.

Second, the Three Core Process model helps to promote a patient-focused orientation by visibly aligning processes and improvement efforts toward the needs of the patient. The conceptual view of operations and administration are always in the context of how the patient moves through the entire system to access a clinical process. For example, a seemingly simple supervisory decision such as scheduling lunch breaks took on new meaning for one emergency department when the decision was viewed based on patient flow. Although scheduling staff to have their lunch breaks at noon seemed reasonable, this practice created unnecessary patient delays and bottlenecks in the patient care processes because patient visits for follow-up care typically increased during the hours of 11:00 a.m. to 1:00 p.m. If the department's focus was the patients, then staff should be present when patients needed them. As a result, the break policy was revised so staff breaks occurred before and after—rather than during—busy patient times.

Third, the model reinforces the different yet necessary and interdependent contributions that each core process and the providers/implementers of those processes provide to patient care and organizational outcomes. This way, collaboration between the entire care team can be promoted, as one administrator told a group of physicians: "I am not going to tell you how to practice medicine. However, it is important that I know your needs so that you may deliver quality care, and you need to know the constraints I am under to provide you with what you need. The best decisions will come by working and planning together."

Fourth, when the administrative role is viewed as a process rather than a function or a structure, all of the tools used to improve other types of processes may also be applied to administrative processes to assist managers in improving their own effectiveness. If one of the desired outcomes is patient satisfaction, the administrative decision-making processes must include mechanisms to collect, analyze, report, communicate, and evaluate patient satisfaction data on a regular basis.

Socioecological Framework

The Socioecological Framework is a systems perspective on promoting health that comes from the field of health behavior and health education (HBHE). This field uses and reflects theory from many disciplines, including psychology, sociology, political science, education, cultural anthropology, biostatistics, epidemiology, health policy, and business administration. The Socioecological Framework, in turn, provides an integrated and multidisciplinary systems perspective of health and health behaviors (Reed 2001).

The Socioecological Framework shown in Figure 5.3 illustrates the four levels of determinants of health behavior: individual, organization, community, and population (Reed 2001; Stokols 1992). For example, determinants of smoking behavior may be described according to the different levels:

1. Individual: a person's knowledge of health risks associated with smoking influences behavior.
2. Organization: the availability of smoking cessation classes as an employee health benefit influences behavior.
3. Community: social norms and beliefs (that is, if smoking is linked to a certain social status) influence behavior.

FIGURE 5.3

Socio-
ecological
Framework

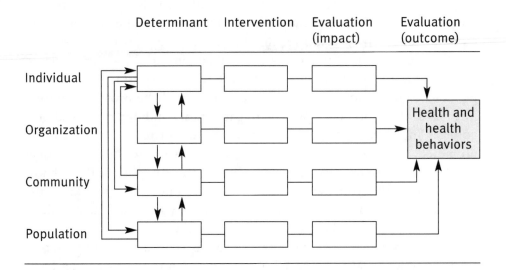

Source: Reprinted with permission by JoAnne Earp, Sc.D.; Peter Reed, M.P.H.; and the instructors of HBHE 131, *Introduction to Social Behavior in Public Health,* Department of Health Behavior and Health Education, University of North Carolina at Chapel Hill, School of Public Health, 2001.

4. Population: regulations that limit smoking in public buildings influence behavior.

In the figure, the arrows pointing to the levels indicate the interconnectedness of these levels as they influence health and health behaviors. As the Socioecological Framework figure shows, interventions and
the evaluation of their impact may be level specific, but they also interact
to influence health and health behavior outcomes.

Lessons for Healthcare Managers

The major lesson from this model for healthcare managers is that it provides a more expansive view of the nature of health in general and of healthcare delivery specifically. In doing so, the model offers a larger context
from which to understand improvement interventions targeted at individuals (e.g., physicians) and organizations (e.g., hospitals).

The other lesson from the Socioecological Framework is that it clearly
illustrates that the interactions between the four levels ultimately influence
health outcomes. This understanding promotes creating comprehensive
interventions within and between levels when appropriate. For example,
since the publication of the Institute of Medicine (2000) report, *To Err Is
Human,* the topic of medical errors has been receiving increasing attention in the lay, professional, and policy communities. An understanding of

the Socioecological Framework will encourage managers to find out why interventions designed to encourage physicians to participate in identifying, reporting, and reducing errors in the clinical practice environment may or may not be effective. Issues at the state and policy levels related to topics such as disclosure; privilege; contract and tort law; and industry regulations, such as JCAHO requirements (Liang 1999, 2000; Liang and Cullen 1999), will also influence participation in well-intended solutions aimed at individual and organizational levels.

Even though a healthcare manager may not be responsible for policy decisions, his or her awareness of the interaction of the levels in the Socioecological Framework can provide the impetus and direction for establishing community partnerships and evaluating intended and unintended consequences of quality interventions within the manager's own organization.

The Baldrige National Quality Program Healthcare Criteria for Performance Excellence

The Baldrige National Quality Program (BNQP) Healthcare Criteria for Performance Excellence provide the most contemporary framework for organizational effectiveness as described in Chapter 1 (Dean and Bowen 1994). For readers who desire a more in-depth explanation, a complete version of these criteria may be found on the Baldrige web site at www.baldrige.gov (Baldrige National Quality Program 2003).

Figure 5.4 illustrates the essential elements in the model and the links between these elements. The following description explains how to read and interpret the figure:

> Your organizational profile (top of figure) sets the context for the way your organization operates. Your environment, key working relationships, and strategic challenges serve as an overarching guide for your organizational performance management system.
>
> The system operations are composed of the six Baldrige categories in the center of the figure that define your operations and the results you can achieve. Leadership; Strategic Planning; and Focus on Patients, Other Customers, and Markets represent the leadership triad. These categories are placed together to emphasize the importance of a leadership focus on strategy and patients/customers. Senior leaders set your organizational direction and seek future opportunities for your organization. Staff Focus, Process Management, and Organizational Performance Results represent the results triad. Your organization's staff and its key processes accomplish the work of the organization that yields your performance results.

FIGURE 5.4

Baldrige
Healthcare
Criteria for
Performance
Excellence
Framework

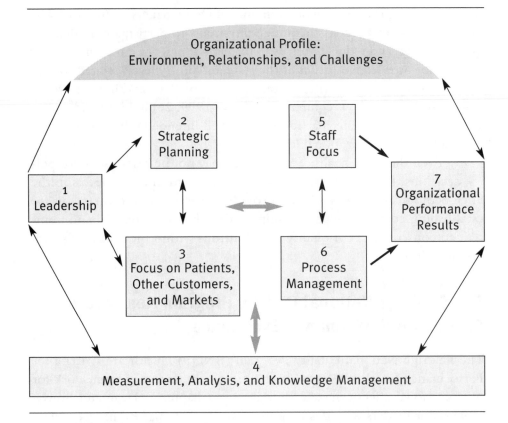

Source: Baldrige National Quality Program. 2003. "Criteria for Performance Excellence." [Online information; retrieved 2/15/03]. http://www.baldrige.gov/Healthcare_Criteria.2002.htm.

All actions point toward Organizational Performance Results—a composite of healthcare, patient and other customer financial, and internal operational performance results, including staff and work system results and social responsibility results. The horizontal arrow in the center of the framework links the leadership triad to the results triad, a linkage critical to organizational success. Furthermore, the arrow indicates the central relationship between Leadership and Organizational Performance Results. The two-headed arrow indicates the importance of feedback in an effective performance management system.

Measurement, Analysis and Knowledge Management are critical to the effective management of your organization and to a fact-based system for improving healthcare and operational performance. Measurement, analysis, and knowledge serve as a foundation for the performance management system. (National Institute of Standards and Technology 2003)

Lessons for Healthcare Managers

Managers may take several lessons from this BNQP systems model. First, the model describes the essential elements for organizational effectiveness (represented by the seven boxes in the model) and how they are related. When viewed in light of the BNQP model, one can see that the principles of total quality, described in Chapter 2, (i.e., customer focus, continuous improvement, and teamwork) address some required elements (i.e., focus on patients, other customers, and markets; process management; and staff focus) but not all of the required elements. The BNQP model suggests that quality management, as defined in Chapter 1, in a healthcare organization requires managers to focus attention not only on the three principles of total quality but also on how leadership, strategic planning, measurement, analysis and knowledge, and a broader focus on staff contribute to achieving the desired organizational performance results.

For example, managers who use this model understand the link between the elements of process management and staff focus. Before implementing a process improvement, managers would ask themselves, "What needs to happen to ensure that the staff will succeed at implementing the new process?" As a result, managers may need to overstaff when a new process is initially implemented to give employees some leeway as they learn the new process or their new roles. Adapting to something new takes time, and by planning ahead, the manager may be able to negotiate for the short-term budget or productivity variances required for the transition period. An understanding of the BNQP model helps managers realize that their role in process improvement also includes ensuring that employees have the information, training, and tools they need so that they may successfully implement improvements in the work setting.

Second, the BNQP model also illustrates the importance of alignment within the organization. This means that the activities within each box in the model are directed toward achieving the same results and that organizational and management choices are consistent with the organization's mission, vision, values, strategic direction, and patient and stakeholder requirements. For example, one healthcare delivery system offered comprehensive quality improvement training for its managers. Each manager was expected to design and carry out an improvement project as a requirement of the training so each selected a topic on which to focus his or her improvement project. Although each manager demonstrated improvement in the chosen area, the collective improvements of all of the training participants may not have necessarily contributed to the overall organizational objectives. This observation was illustrated by one manager who devoted much time and effort to improve a service area that was eliminated by the organization the following year. Another healthcare organization offering a similar type of training for managers used senior leaders to assist the managers in selecting improvement topics that would not only provide benefit within the manager's scope of responsibility but also contribute to the overall organizational goals.

Third, this model illustrates the importance of alignment of data, analysis, and performance indicators. Managers using the BNQP model would choose performance indicators in a systematic way. When designing their performance measurement system and selecting performance indicators, managers may consistently ask themselves the following series of questions (National Institute of Standards and Technology 2003):

- What are the key determinants of success for our setting of care?
- Who are our patients and stakeholders, and what are their requirements?
- How do these determinants and requirements guide decisions about our organizational goals?
- Are these goals consistent with the mission, vision, and values of the organization?
- What approach(es) will we use to meet our goals?
- What is the desired impact for selecting this particular approach?
- What performance indicators will allow us to measure the desired impact?
- How often should each of these indicators be reviewed, and by whom?
- What data collection, analysis, and reporting capabilities are necessary to deliver the performance indicators as determined?

Finally, the BNQP model provides the manager a vehicle for initiating and continuing discussions about performance excellence within the organization.

Conclusion

This chapter presents four different systems models for managers. Table 5.1 summarizes key lessons for managers in each of these models. Whichever model the manager chooses to use, the common benefit of using systems models is that they encourage the manager to do the following:

- broaden his or her perspective to see his or her own work environment, department, and organization within a larger context;
- better understand the interconnectedness and relationships between various components within an organization that contribute to performance results; and
- realize that results are achieved by design, that design is a choice, and that to achieve better results, managers must improve the quality of their choices.

OSD Model	TCP Model	Socio-ecological Model	BNQP
Empowers managers to make different choices about how the system operates Recognizes behavior and feelings as system outputs	Improves interdependent processes concurrently Aligns processes around patient needs Values all provider and employee groups Views administrative role as a process rather than a function	Broadens and expands the manager's view Addresses community and policy influences on health outcomes	Shows how the components of performance excellence are related Promotes alignment of all activities within the organization Promotes alignment of performance indicators Enhances communication around performance excellence

TABLE 5.1
Systems Models: Lessons for Managers

The exercise at the end of this chapter provides an opportunity to use the systems models to better understand how organizational relationships influence quality. Chapter 6 addresses another aspect of the systems approach: the concept of systemic structure in organizations.

Companion Readings

Baldrige National Quality Program. 2003. "Healthcare Criteria for Performance Excellence." [Online information; retrieved 2/15/03]. http://www.baldrige.gov/Criteria.htm.
Kelly, D. L., S. L. Pestotnik, M. C. Coons, and J. W. Lelis. 1997. "Reengineering a Surgical Service Line: Focusing on Core Process Improvement." *American Journal of Medical Quality* 12 (2): 120–29.

References

Axtell, R. N., and S. L. Eckholdt. 1992. "Organizational Systems Design: Enriching Lives by Creating Self-Designing Organizations" Workshop. Presented by the Alliance of Organizational System Designers, Snowbird, Utah, September 23–25.

Baldrige National Quality Program. 2003. "Healthcare Criteria for Performance Excellence." [Online information; retrieved 2/15/03]. http://www.baldrige.gov/Criteria.htm.

———. 2001. "1999 Award Recipients Applications Summaries." [Online information; retrieved 2/15/03]. http://www.baldrige.gov/1999_Application_Summaries.htm.

Dean, J. W., and D. E. Bowen. 1994. "Management Theory and Total Quality: Improving Research and Practice through Theory Development." *Academy of Management Review* 19 (2): 392–418.

Institute of Medicine. 2000. *To Err Is Human: Building a Safer Health System.* Washington, DC: National Academy Press.

Kelly, D. L., S. L. Pestotnik, M. C. Coons, and J. W. Lelis. 1997. "Reengineering a Surgical Service Line: Focusing on Core Process Improvement." *American Journal of Medical Quality* 12 (2): 120–29.

Liang, B. A. 2000. "Creating Problems as Part of the 'Solution': The JCAHO Sentinel Event Policy, Legal Issues and Patient Safety." *Journal of Health Law* 33 (2): 263–85.

———. 1999. "Error in Medicine: Legal Impediments to U.S. Reform." *Journal of Health Politics, Policy and Law* 24 (1): 27–58.

Liang, B. A., and D. J. Cullen. 1999. "The Legal System and Patient Safety: Charting a Divergent Course. The Relationship Between Malpractice Litigation and Human Errors." *Anesthesiology* 91 (3): 609–11.

National Institute of Standards and Technology. 2003. *Baldrige National Quality Program Healthcare Criteria for Performance Excellence.* Gaithersburg, MD: National Institute of Standards and Technology.

Nelson, E. C., J. J. Mohr, P. B. Batalden, and S. K. Plume. 1996. "Improving Healthcare, Part 1: The Clinical Value Compass." *Joint Commission Journal on Quality Improvement* 22 (4): 243–58.

Ostroff, F., and D. Smith. 1992. "The Horizontal Corporation: It's About Managing Across, Not Up and Down." *The McKinsey Quarterly* 1992 (1): 148–68.

Reed, P. 2001. "Introduction to Social Behavior in Public Health." Course lecture at the Department of Health Behavior and Health Education, University of North Carolina at Chapel Hill, School of Public Health.

Stokols, D. 1992. "Establishing and Maintaining Healthy Environments: Toward a Social Ecology of Health Promotion." *American Psychologist* 47 (1): 6–22.

Exercise

Objective: To practice identifying relationships within systems

Instructions:

1. Review the four systems models presented in this chapter:
    *   OSD Model
    *   Three Core Process Model
    *   Socioecological Model
    *   BNQP Healthcare Criteria for Performance Excellence Model
2. Choose one that you can best relate to at this time.
3. Review your responses to the Chapter 1 Exercise. Look at both your excellent quality experience and your poor quality experience, paying particular attention to how you described the manager's role or influence.
4. Now, think about those experiences from the perspective of the systems model you chose in #2. Describe any additional understanding of the experience that you may have when viewing it from a systems perspective, then write your responses in a table similar to the one below.

Systems Model Worksheet

	Manager's role/ influence	Additional understanding by viewing through systems perspective
Excellent quality experience		
Poor quality experience		

SYSTEMIC STRUCTURE

Objectives

- To introduce the metaphor of an iceberg to assist in understanding the concept of systemic structure in organizations
- To discuss practical lessons for healthcare managers resulting from understanding the concept of systemic structure
- To introduce strategies to assist managers in identifying and understanding systemic structures
- To practice identifying different mental models or assumptions in healthcare and understanding how they influence behavior

On Thursday, Nurse Smith volunteered to work a double shift in the intensive care unit (ICU). The next day, she missed her regularly scheduled shift when she called in sick. The following month, Nurse Jones, who works in the same ICU, volunteered to work a double shift. Two days later, she missed her regularly scheduled shift when she called in sick. When the ICU manager mentioned this "coincidence" to her colleagues, they also described similar situations on their respective units. As the ICU manager gathered more information about employee staffing practices, she realized that, although the policies helped staffing in the short term, the same policies were inadvertently contributing to increased sick calls and more overtime in the long run.

The manager was discovering that well-intended efforts, such as the carefully written policies and procedures, may not yield expected results. Likewise, well-intended change or improvement interventions often yield disappointing results. This chapter begins to explore how a systems perspective can help managers improve the quality of organizational interventions.

A Systems Metaphor for Organizations

Metaphors can be a valuable tool because they provide a concrete picture of a theoretical concept (Armenakis and Bedian 1992; Clearly and Packard 1992); after the concept has been translated into a tangible form, it becomes easier to understand and remember. Thinking of an organization as an iceberg is one metaphor that illustrates the subtle but powerful systems principles at work in organizations (Innovation Associates, Inc. 1995). Like an iceberg, where nine-tenths of the iceberg's mass is under water (GLAC-IER 2003), the essence of an organization's makeup is not visible to most observers. Those forces that cause an organization to function the way it does and the people in the organization to behave the way they do may not be readily observable. Yet, just as the part of the iceberg that is beneath the water's surface is dangerous to passing ships, what is below the organizational "waterline" can sink well-intended change and improvement efforts.

The triangular shape in Figure 6.1 represents the iceberg, and the wavy, thick line represents the waterline. The tip of the iceberg (the top layer of the triangle) represents the events that occur daily in the organization. The middle layer of the iceberg represents a deeper understanding of the organization as a system by linking events into patterns of behavior. The bottom level of the iceberg, which is under water, represents the deepest understanding of the behavior of the organization as a system. This level represents relationships among variables in the system that cause the events and patterns to occur.

In the staffing example at the beginning of this chapter, the nurse managers observed the nurses working double shifts and calling in sick as independent events on each of their units. However, while comparing notes, they identified a pattern of behavior across three different patient care units. Although the act of identifying patterns is still above the organizational waterline, it is the first step toward systems thinking. The manager began to go below the waterline when she identified relationships between the observations and patterns. By telling a "story" of her discoveries, the relationships and underlying causes of the problems began to emerge. The story was this:

> The hospital policies were supposed to promote adequate staffing and discourage sick calls; however, the day shifts were often overstaffed and the evening and nights shifts were understaffed.
>
> Nurses were paid overtime (time and a half) for working a double shift. When a nurse volunteered for a double shift, she or he was positively perceived as "helpful" and a "team player." The nurse helped out with a short-staffed shift and did not, in turn, cause a short-staffed shift by calling in sick.
>
> By working a double shift and calling in sick later in the week, the nurses were able to work the same amount of hours but get paid for four extra hours than if they had worked their regularly scheduled shifts.

The manager was beginning to see the relationships among the key variables in the system: scheduling policies, individual employee incentives, compensation and rewards, sick-call policy, individual unit operations, and float pool operations. Although individually, the policies and operations seemed reasonable, their interactions with each other contributed to the

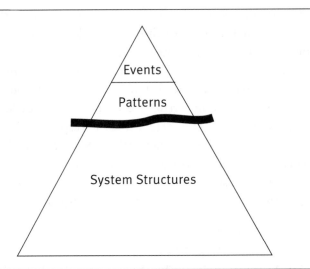

FIGURE 6.1
The Iceberg
Metaphor

Source: Reprinted with permission from Innovations Associates, Inc. 1995. "Systems Thinking: A Language for Learning and Action." Participant manual, version 95.4.1. Waltham, Massachusetts.

underlying systemic structure: the relationship between the perceived benefit to nurses (i.e., helping out peers and patients, earning the same money while working fewer hours, or earning more money while working the same hours) and the frequency of the behavior of volunteering for a double shift and calling in sick later in the week. These two variables were related in a way that reinforced the behavior—that is, as the number of nurses who perceived this benefit increased, the number of times the behavior occurred increased. Note that the nurses had no malicious intent in this case; they were simply following the policies as they were crafted. As this reinforcing relationship occurred across several nursing departments, however, the unintended result to the hospital was an overall increase in salary expense.

Only when the manager understood each of the policies within the context of how they comprised the whole were she and other managers able to redesign the system to achieve the intended result of staffing the hospital in a dependable and cost-effective manner. Some of the changes this organization made to break the reinforcing cycle included reviewing the distribution of nurses during the day, evening, and night shifts to better balance staffing across the 24-hour period; improving coordination between the nursing unit schedules and the float pool's schedules; and changing the overtime criteria (consistent with legal labor requirements) from hours worked in excess of eight hours per day to hours worked in excess of 40 hours per week.

Lessons for Healthcare Managers

When using the iceberg metaphor to describe an organization, events and patterns may be thought of as occurring above the waterline. The term *systemic structure* refers to what is found below the waterline. Systemic structure involves the interrelationships among key variables within the system and the influence of these interrelationships on the system's behavior over time (Senge 1990). Note that systemic structure refers to interrelationships among variables in the system and not to interpersonal relationships among people. Systemic structure should also be differentiated from *organizational structure,* which refers to how responsibility and authority are distributed throughout an organization (Shortell and Kaluzny 2000).

Valuable insights about organizations may be gained by understanding the concept of systemic structure. This section offers four lessons for healthcare managers that have resulted from these insights:

1.   Systemic structure influences behavior
2.   Systemic structure is invisible
3.   Information is essential to identifying systemic structure
4.   Successful change requires going below the waterline

Lesson 1: Systemic Structure Influences Behavior

Consider the following story from an anonymous author:

> A college student spent an entire summer going to the football field every day wearing a black-and-white striped shirt, walking up and down the field for ten or fifteen minutes, throwing bird seed all over the field, blowing a whistle, and then walking off the field. At the end of the summer, it came time for the first home football game. The referee walked onto the field and blew the whistle. The game had to be delayed for a half hour to wait for the birds to get off the field.

We all laugh at this story. However, if we were sitting in the stadium stands without a clue about the events of the summer, we would probably be annoyed and blame those darn birds. The birds were not right or wrong. They were doing exactly what they were supposed to be doing based on the underlying systemic structures: the relationships between feeding time and the football field, the striped shirt and the bird seed, the whistle and their hunger. Similar situations occur with providers and employees in healthcare organizations. The thought of a healthcare professional coming to work to intentionally do a poor job seems absurd. However, the desire to blame is often an initial management response to a negative situation or a negative outcome.

"Every organization is perfectly designed to get the results that it gets. To get different result you need to improve the design of the organization" (Hanna 1988). This expression has become a common phrase in quality improvement presentations and articles. However, what is not commonly heard or read is that design needs to be improved not only above the waterline but below the waterline as well. The phrase "every organization is perfectly designed to get the results that is gets" is usually applied within the context of events (i.e., the top level of the iceberg). When improvements are designed from the event level, managers and providers will typically ask, "What do we need to *do* differently? What *actions* (e.g., implementing clinical guidelines, streamlining office scheduling systems, installing new computers) will bring us closer to our vision of quality healthcare?"

An understanding of the iceberg metaphor, however, shows us that questions must be asked from all levels of the iceberg, from observing events to determining patterns in the events to identifying underlying structures that cause the patterns and events to occur. This changing view also alters the questions the managers and providers must ask. Rather than focusing only on "What can we *do* differently?" managers must also ask, "How can we best *understand why* we are getting the results we are getting?" The manager will then begin to look for patterns in recurrent events, to try to understand how past events may be contributing to current behavior, and to begin to uncover the key relationships among variables that are influencing current behavior of the system. Only when this has been done can the manager target interventions that alter these relationships and that in turn lead to sustainable improvements in the actions intended to deliver better organizational and patient results.

Lesson 2: Systemic Structure Is Invisible

Systemic structure is usually invisible unless we make a conscious effort to find it. As with an iceberg, just because managers do not see what is below the organizational waterline does not mean that systemic structure is not present in the organization. For example, a newly hired manager at an academic medical center was assigned to facilitate an improvement project on one patient care unit. If the project proved successful on this unit, the intent was to expand the intervention organizationwide. Despite positive results, as measured by reduced cycle times, increased patient satisfaction, and increased staff satisfaction, the project was not implemented beyond the original pilot site. When the manager began to explore possible reasons that the project was not replicated on the other units, he discovered that over the years numerous project teams had designed and implemented successful pilot projects aimed at improving specific problems. However, very few of these projects had actually been integrated into the ongoing activities of the organization (i.e., institutionalized).

Upon further investigation, he uncovered the following systemic structures operating in this organization. First, all improvements in the organization were called "pilots." The expectation was that a trial would be conducted for a specified period of time, that results would be presented to the administrative team, and that the administrative team would then authorize the project to continue or not. The problem was that this process occurred independently from the budgeting process. When the "special pools" of dollars to fund a pilot were gone, no mechanisms were in place to reallocate funds either within or among departments to support a successful improvement or innovation.

The pilot label also brought with it other short-term perceptions related to support, staffing, and budgets. Because of these invisible, but real, relationships among the variables required to support change, this academic medical center demonstrated a constant stream of successful improvement pilot efforts yet wondered why sustained improvement in the overall organizational performance never occurred.

Lesson 3: Information Is Essential to Identifying Systemic Structure

A *pattern* is "a consistent, characteristic form, style, or method; composite of traits or features characteristic of an individual or a group" (Dictionary.com 2003). This definition implies that identifying or recognizing a pattern requires more than one observation. In the nurse manager example, the discussion among the nurse managers about issues on their respective units provided an opportunity to observe behavior of many nurses across multiple units. Only when these observations were combined did the organizational pattern become evident.

The need for multiple observations or data points has implications for how managers determine organizational structure, interact and communicate, and present performance data. The traditional vertical organizational structure, which compartmentalizes groups within rigid reporting lines, reduces the opportunity to interact across departments and disciplines and reduces the opportunity to identify organizational patterns. Communication methods based on "telling" rather than "sharing" information also reduce the opportunity to identify organizational patterns by reducing two-way communication and the "fresh eyes" often needed to interpret and link events. Data reported by single time periods only (e.g., monthly departmental financial reports) reduce managers' ability to identify patterns over time in their own departments, while aggregated, organizational data reduce managers' opportunity to identify patterns across smaller units of analysis within the organization.

Strategies that can promote pattern identification and prompt investigation into underlying structures include

- organizational structures and/or culture that encourage interaction among levels and units;
- open and free flow of information; and
- displaying performance data on run charts or control charts to make data trends over time more visible (Chapter 9 further explores the role of measurement in pattern identification).

Lesson 4: Successful Change Requires Going Below the Waterline

To implement successful and lasting change efforts, managers must go below the organizational waterline. An understanding of the iceberg metaphor explains why the potential of many change or improvement efforts are not fully realized. If changes are targeted at the event or pattern levels (i.e., what we do) rather than at the systemic structure level (i.e., what causes the system to behave the way it does), the impact will only be temporary. Because structure influences behavior, the only way to truly change behavior within the system is to identify, target, and change the underlying structures.

There is no shortage of ideas on how to improve our organizational systems; however, a common challenge for managers and care providers alike is how to actually implement these ideas. Organizational culture may be thought of as an underlying systemic structure. The influence of hospital culture on the ability to convert continuous quality improvement concepts into effective implementation has been described in the healthcare research literature (Shortell et al. 1995). Another example may be seen in the area of clinical practice guidelines. Although providers generally support evidence-based practice, translating evidence into practice has been difficult to achieve (Cabana et al. 1999; Solberg 2002). The clinical literature is now addressing the relationship of systemic structures, such as leadership, context, and incentives, to guideline implementation (McCormack et al. 2002; Solberg 2000a, 2000b).

Going Below the Waterline

A captain of a ship sailing in the North Atlantic uses radar, a sonar, and a bow watch (a sailor posted at the front of the ship to look out for danger) to alert him to underwater ice. Likewise, managers may also use strategies that alert them to underlying systemic structures. Three strategies that managers may use are

1. understanding history,
2. being aware of mental models, and
3. integrating double-loop learning into their management philosophy and approach.

Understanding History

History is a powerful underlying structure. A healthcare manager's current work may be influenced by the department's history, the hospital's history, a professional group's history, the community's history, or the industry's history. For example, the sudden death of a well-respected department manager had a long-lasting impact on the department staff. The new incumbent manager was faced not only with getting settled in a new role and new department but also with addressing the staff's grief. For new employees, the lack of shared history with the deceased manager was a source of polarization between the "before" and "after" staff and interfered with the entire staff's ability to achieve a high level of teamwork.

A nurse at a rehabilitation center that had recently been purchased by a "for-profit" organization carefully explained the organization's history to a patient's family. The previous owners and managers of the center were proud of their heritage of religious service and quality. The family inquired if their family member would still get what she needed at this for-profit facility, and the nurse informed the family that the staff still identified with the center's historic values.

In the book *The Social Transformation of American Medicine,* Paul Starr (1982) describes the evolution of the American medical profession and physicians' roles from the eighteenth through the twentieth century. Although one may agree or disagree with Starr's conclusions, this book explains how the history of physicians, hospitals, and insurance companies shaped the healthcare industry of today, and as such the book provides a level of understanding of the current state of our healthcare system. Understanding the circumstances surrounding the Flexner report, which was published in 1910 and describes the state of medical education at the time, can provide insights into why medical schools are structured the way they are and into the role of academic medical centers in U.S. healthcare. Understanding the numerous occasions that national health insurance has been on the political agenda (1917, the 1930s, and the 1940s) as well as the American Medical Association's role in those debates can provide insight into physicians' responses to contemporary issues surrounding healthcare reform (Starr 1982).

The simplest strategies that managers may use to understand history are to ask, listen, and read. In addition, approaches to large-group "visioning" meetings have incorporated structured discussions about history (Weisbord 1987). Managers, especially those assuming a new role, may gain valuable insights by facilitating similar discussions with staff in their own departments. The following guidelines may help:

- Ask the group to identify significant events during defined periods of time. Events within the department, organization, community, clinical specialty or profession, or industry may be identified.
- List the events by periods of time (e.g., in five- or ten-year increments, depending on the group).
- Look for patterns in the listed events.

Examples of Group Discussions

One group of nurses in the postpartum area identified this event in their history discussion: at 5:00 every morning, the charge nurse would announce over the unit's intercom system: "Patients who have not had a bowel movement yet, please put on your nurse call light." The group burst into laughter, and one nurse observed, "Glad those 'good old days' are gone!" This simple observation helped the group to let go of its resistance to a proposed change on the unit as it realized that it had experienced numerous changes over the years, most of which had direct benefit to the patients.

A manager in a laboratory was intrigued about the type of events identified during the history discussion with staff. Most of the identified events focused on current events from the news, and few events focused on laboratory technology or the department, as he had anticipated. What this manager realized was that because the demographic composition of his department had been changing over the years (the technologists were 40 years old or older, the technical assistants and phlebotomists were 30 years old or younger), the two distinct demographics had little in common to talk about but current events. This realization not only helped to explain why previous team-building sessions had only been moderately successful but also prompted the manager to establish common ground for his employees through a shared vision for the department. This manager also became more attentive to age diversity, succession planning, and the needs of differing demographic groups, particularly in his approaches to recruitment and hiring (Kelly 1999).

Being Aware of Mental Models

The term *mental model* is often used interchangeably with the terms "paradigm" and "assumption." Although these terms are technically slightly different, they all refer to a deeply ingrained way of thinking that influences how a person sees and understands the world as well as how that person acts. When someone declares an unquestionable status or condition, a mental model is usually being expressed; words like "always" and "never" are clues that mental models are being expressed. Mental models may be so strong that they override the facts at hand. For example, at a quality management workshop, one hospital manager stated her mental model as follows: "Physicians would never spend time at a workshop like this." However, sitting beside her for the duration of the workshop were two pediatricians and a family practitioner!

What this manager did not realize was that her own mental model was interfering with her ability to design appropriate strategies to engage physicians in improvement efforts in her own organization. As a result of her mental model, she found numerous reasons why physicians would not participate and was blinded to strategies to encourage physician participation. To promote learning and improvement in organizations, managers, care providers, and other employees in the organization must "look inward . . . to reflect critically on their own behavior, identify ways they often inadvertently contribute to the organization's problems, and then change how they act" (Argyris 1991). Without an understanding of our own mental models, we run the risk of unknowingly undermining our own efforts to progress along the quality continuum.

Differing mental models may also be a source of conflict within the organization. A manager's view or perspective on organizations themselves will shape his or her management strategies, actions, and style. Two contrasting views of organizations are the *rational model* and *political model*, which are shown in Table 6.1 and illustrated in the following example.

A manager who viewed organizations through a rational model was extremely frustrated with and ineffective in an organization that operated from a political perspective. From the manager's point of view, the decision-making processes in this politically driven organization served the interest of the players involved but did not result in optimal patient outcomes or cost-effective approaches. On the other hand, the administrative team perceived this manager's emphasis on results as interfering with the delicate political alliances they had worked very hard to establish. The lack of understanding of each other's mental models created ongoing conflict between the manager and administrative team: the manager thought that the team did not care about results, and the team thought that the manager was compromising relationships with important stakeholders. Without an awareness of each other's mental models, the conflict between the manager and the administrators continued to grow until the manager finally left the organization.

Had both parties made their mental models explicit—whether through discussion, definition of organizational operating principles, or orientation of new managers to the culture of decision making—their conflict may have been avoided or at least some common understanding may have been established. Instead, the results were conflict; tension; and, eventually, manager turnover.

Integrating Double-Loop Learning

In one large hospital, a nursing supervisor complained to the manager of environmental services that when the housekeeper was asked to move a piece of equipment to prepare a room for a patient admission, the housekeeper refused to do so. The supervisor accused the housekeeper of being uncooperative and an obstacle to patient care. The supervisor operated from a professional mindset and believed that the housekeeper should be able to determine when the medical equipment may be touched. Because of language, cultural, and educational differences among staff in entry-level positions, the environmental services staff needed to strictly adhere to the department's standard policies and procedures. The housekeeper was operating from one set of assumptions (i.e., following the rules by not touching the nurses' equipment), while the nursing supervisor was operating from a conflicting set of assumptions (i.e., doing whatever needs to be done

Organizational Characteristic	Rational Model	Political Model
Goals, preferences	Consistent across members	Inconsistent, pluralistic within the organization
Power and control	Centralized	Diffuse, shifting coalitions and interest groups
Decision process	Logical, orderly, sequential	Disorderly, give and take of competing interests
Information	Extensive, systematic, accurate	Ambiguous, selectively available, used as a power resource
Cause-and-effect relationships	Predictable	Uncertain
Decisions	Based on outcome-maximizing choice	Results from bargaining and interplay among interests
Ideology	Efficiency and effectiveness	Struggle, conflict, winners and losers

TABLE 6.1
Comparison of Organizational Models

Source: From *Health Care Management: Organization Design and Behavior,* 4th edition, by S. M. Shortell and A. D. Kaluzny. © 2000. Reprinted with permission of Delmar Learning, a division of Thomson Learning: www.thomsonrights.com. Fax 800 730-2215.

to care for the patient). Although both parties were trying to do their jobs the best way they knew how, their opposing assumptions led to conflict and antagonism between the two departments.

This situation of "accidental adversaries" may be unintentionally created when underlying assumptions are not known. The numerous roles, backgrounds, personalities, levels of education, and other diverse characteristics of the healthcare workforce necessitate managers to use double-loop learning as a valuable strategy to promote teamwork and quality within their scope of responsibility. *Double-loop learning* occurs when underlying assumptions are examined and when subsequent action, based on what the assumptions reveal, is taken (Argyris 1991). In the workplace, however, managers unfortunately often spend more time trying to mend adversarial relationships than preventing them. Managers may minimize accidental adversaries by

- clarifying operating principles,
- helping staff understand and communicate its own assumptions,
- helping staff ask for clarification and explanations of others' behavior, and

- explicitly describing their (managers) own expectations for individual employees and for teams.

Double-loop learning is not appropriate for all situations in a health-care organization. For example, in the middle of an emergency resuscitation is not the time to question why a cardiac arrest code is carried out in a certain manner. As described in Chapter 1, efficiency and consistency in day-to-day operations is accomplished through minimizing variation in how processes are carried out. However, double-loop learning should be an integral part of efforts that require innovative solutions or that require improved levels of performance. Managers and teams should be comfortable with asking themselves and others questions such as, "Why do we do things the way we do? Is there a better way to get the job done? Are my own mental models helping or hurting my and our team's/department's/ organization's effectiveness?"

For an improvement team, double-loop learning may take the form of discussions that question "whether operating norms are appropriate—then inventing new norms as needed" (Pierce 2000). Innovative solutions (e.g., open-access scheduling) result from the process of double-loop learning. This type of scheduling approach, which is used by pediatricians and family practitioners, challenges operating norms and assumptions around outpatient scheduling (Randolph and Lannon 2001; Tumolo 2002). Managers may consider assigning a team member to be the "devil's advocate" to ensure that assumptions are tested and challenged; otherwise, the challenger may be viewed as a barrier to the team process.

Conclusion

This chapter introduces the concept of systemic structure in organizations and explores lessons and strategies for managers. If managers and organizations are to achieve new levels of performance, managers must begin to integrate double-loop learning into their philosophy and approaches. The exercise at the end of this chapter provides an opportunity to explore how mental models influence managers' behavior and to analyze an accidental adversaries relationship. Section 3 of this book challenges assumptions around some common management operating norms and presents a new set of norms that enhance an individual's ability to operate from a quality management perspective.

Companion Readings

Kelly, D. L. 1998. "Reframing Beliefs About Work and Change Processes in Redesigning Laboratory Services." *Joint Commission Journal on Quality Improvement* 24 (9): 154–67.

Starr, P. 1982. *The Social Transformation of American Medicine: The Rise of a Sovereign Profession and the Making of a Vast Industry,* 235–89. Reading, MA: The Perseus Books Group.

References

Argyris, C. 1991. "Teaching Smart People How to Learn." *Harvard Business Review* 69 (3): 99–110.

Armenakis, A. A., and A. G. Bedian. 1992. "The Role of Metaphors in Organizational Change." *Group and Organizational Management* 17 (3): 242–48.

Cabana, M. D., C. S. Rand, N. R. Powe, A. W. Wu, M. H. Wilson, P. A. Abboud, and H. R. Rubin. 1999. "Why Don't Physicians Follow Clinical Practice Guidelines? A Framework for Improvement." *Journal of the American Medical Association* 282 (15): 1458–65.

Clearly, C., and T. Packard. 1992. "The Use of Metaphors in Organizational Assessment and Change." *Group and Organizational Management* 17 (3): 229–41.

Dictionary.com. 2003. "Dictionary.com home page." [Online information; retrieved 2/16/03]. http://www.dictionary.com.

GLACIER. 2003. "GLACIER home page." [Online information; retrieved 2/16/03]. http://www.glacier.rice.edu.

Hanna, D. P. 1988. *Designing Organizations for High Performance.* Reading, MA: Addison-Wesley Publishing Company.

Innovations Associates, Inc. 1995. "Systems Thinking: A Language for Learning and Action." Participant manual, version 95.4.1. Waltham, MA: Innovations Associates, Inc.

Kelly, D. L. 1999. "Systems Thinking: A Tool for Organizational Diagnosis in Healthcare." In *Making it Happen: Stories from Inside the New Workplace,* compiled from *The Systems Thinker Newsletter,* 1989–97. Waltham, MA: Pegasus Communications, Inc.

McCormack, B., A. Kitson, G. Harvey, J. Rycroft-Malone, A. Titchen, and K. Seers. 2002. "Getting Evidence into Practice: The Meaning of 'Context'." *Journal of Advanced Nursing* 38 (1): 94–104.

Pierce, J. C. 2000. "The Paradox of Physicians and Administrators in Healthcare Organizations." *Healthcare Management Review* 25 (1): 7–28.

Randolph, G., and C. Lannon. 2001. "Advanced Access Scheduling: Doing Today's Work Today." *American Academy of Pediatrics News* 19 (6): 266.

Schein, E. H. 1992. *Organizational Culture and Leadership.* San Francisco: Jossey-Bass.

Senge, P. M. 1990. *The Fifth Discipline: The Art and Practice of the Learning Organization.* New York: Doubleday Currency.

Shortell, S. M., and A. D. Kaluzny. 2000. *Healthcare Management: Organization Design and Behavior.* Albany, NY: Delmar Thomson Learning.

Shortell, S. M., J. L. O'Brien, J. M. Carman, R. W. Foster, E. F. X. Hughes, H. Boerstler, and E. J. O'Connor. 1995. "Assessing the Impact of

Continuous Quality Improvement/Total Quality Management: Concept versus Implementation." *Healthcare Research* 30 (2): 377–99.

Solberg, L. I. 2002. "Guideline Implementation: Why Don't We Do it?" *American Family Physician* 65 (2): 176, 181–82.

———. 2000a. "Incentivising, Facilitating and Implementing an Office Tobacco Cessation System." *Tobacco Control* 9 (Suppl 1): i37–41.

———. 2000b. "Lessons from Experienced Guideline Implementers: Attend to Many Factors and Use Multiple Strategies." *Joint Commission Journal on Quality Improvement* 26 (4): 171–88.

Starr, P. 1982. *The Social Transformation of American Medicine: The Rise of a Sovereign Profession and the Making of a Vast Industry.* Reading, MA: The Perseus Books Group.

Tumolo, J. 2002. "Open-Access Scheduling." *Advanced Nurse Practitioner* 10 (5): 25.

Weisbord, M. R. 1987. *Productive Workplaces: Organizing and Managing for Dignity and Community.* San Francisco: Jossey-Bass.

Exercise

Objective: To begin to understand how mental models or assumptions influence behavior in organizations

Instructions:

1. a. See the Mental Models Worksheet below. Identify two different mental models, in the context of a healthcare organization, for each of the categories listed. An example has been provided for the Clinical Guidelines category. Write your responses in the respective boxes on the worksheet.

    b. Describe how each of these mental models would influence your actions and behavior in your role as a healthcare manager. Write your response in the respective boxes on the worksheet.

    c. Choose four mental models (one in each category) that currently influence or that you would like to influence your management approach and style. Circle those mental models on the worksheet.

2. Read the case and respond to the questions afterward.

Case Study

This case is from E. H. Schein. 1992. *Organizational Culture and Leadership.* San Francisco: Jossey-Bass.

Unconscious assumptions sometimes lead to catch-22 situations, as illustrated by a common problem experienced by American supervisors in other cultures. A manager who comes from an American pragmatic tradition assumes and takes for granted that solving a problem always takes the highest priority. When that manager encounters a subordinate who comes from a different cultural background, in which good relationships and protecting the superior's 'face' are assumed to have top priority, the following scenario can easily result.

The manager proposes a solution to a given problem. The subordinate knows that the solution will not work, but his unconscious assumption requires that he remain silent because to tell the boss that the proposed solution is wrong is a threat to the boss's face. The subordinate would not even think to do anything other than to remain silent or even reassure the boss that she should go ahead and take the action.

The action is taken, and the results are negative. The boss, somewhat surprised and puzzled, asks the subordinate what he would have done. When the subordinate reports that he would have done something different, the boss quite legitimately asks why the subordinate did not speak up sooner. This question puts the subordinate in an impossible bind because the answer itself is a threat to the boss's face. He cannot possibly explain his behavior without committing the very sin he is trying to avoid in the first place—namely, embarrassing the boss. He might even lie at this point and argue that what the boss did was right and only bad luck or uncontrollable circumstances prevented it from succeeding.

From the point of view of the subordinate, the boss's behavior is incomprehensible because it shows lack of self-pride, possibly causing the subordinate to lose respect for that boss. To the boss, the subordinate's behavior is equally incomprehensible. She cannot develop any sensible explanation of his subordinate's behavior that is not cynically colored by the assumption that the subordinate at some level just does not care about effective performance and therefore must be fired. The assumption "one never embarrasses a superior" never even occurs to the boss as operating in this case or that the assumption "one gets the job done" is even more powerful for the subordinate.

1. Describe the results of this case when the employee and the boss are operating from opposing mental models.

2. Double-loop learning occurs when underlying assumptions are examined and subsequent action, based on what the assumptions reveal, is taken. Describe an alternative case in which double-loop learning could have been used. How would the employee and the boss have behaved differently? What alternative results could have been achieved?

Mental Models Worksheet

	Mental Model	Actions	Alternative Mental Model	Actions
Clinical Guidelines	Clinical guidelines used to control physician behavior		Using evidence-based clinical guidelines to standardize steps of care can actually save physician time on routine interventions so that more time can be spent on the unique needs of that patient	
Use of Data				
Management/ Physician Relationships				
"Fighting Fires" Management Style				

ACHIEVING QUALITY RESULTS IN COMPLEX SYSTEMS

GOALS

Objectives

- To explore why effective goal setting is essential to quality management
- To gain an appreciation for the relationship between how goals are stated and the ability to obtain desired results
- To contrast different types of goal statements
- To practice setting goals

A guest lecturer, formerly a neonatal intensive care nurse, led health administration doctoral students on a discussion about organizational effectiveness. At the conclusion of the discussion, one student observed that the previous guest lecturer also had a background in pediatrics (Bordley et al. 2001; Margolis et al. 2001). The student asked the lecturer if a relationship existed between an interest in quality and a background in pediatrics. The guest lecturer paused for reflection and then replied, "Maybe it's because we see life at its beginning and understand how important a healthy start to life is."

The same idea can be applied to the setting of goals. A "healthy start" to an improvement effort or management intervention begins with an effective goal. This chapter explores the reason that effective goal setting is essential to quality management, the relationship between goals and results, and the approaches that managers can employ to improve their goal-setting skills.

Importance of Setting Goals

In healthcare organizations, the influence of goals on quality may be seen in both clinical interventions and management interventions.

Clinical Interventions

Patient A presents to his primary care provider as overweight and suffering from high blood pressure. The treatment goals the provider sets for the patient are to lose weight and to take the prescribed blood pressure medicine. The patient begins dieting and taking his blood pressure medicine. Within six months, Patient A has lost 30 pounds and shows improved blood pressure. However, at Patient A's annual checkup several months later, his provider is dismayed to find that Patient A gained back the 30 pounds.

Patient B presents to his primary care provider as overweight and suffering from high blood pressure. The treatment goals the provider sets for the patient are to integrate a balanced diet and regular exercise into the patient's daily lifestyle and to reduce blood pressure through lifestyle change and medication. Within six months, Patient B has also lost 30 pounds and shows improved blood pressure. At his next annual physical, Patient B has kept off the 30 pounds and informs his provider that he feels much better since he has been walking three days a week and eating healthier.

The seemingly subtle difference in how the treatment goals were set for these two patients actually represents the relationship between the goals and the subsequent results that are obtained. Patient A and Patient B both presented with similar situations. Both providers were conscientious and caring and made the appropriate diagnosis. The difference in the impact and sustainability of the interventions was in how the goals were set.

Managerial Interventions

Goals serve many purposes in organizations (Scott 1998); they are integrated into most aspects of a manager's role and functions at all levels of the organization. Goals help a manager to select among many alternative courses of action. For example, for the goal of reducing waiting times in the clinic to improve patient satisfaction, a proposed intervention that would reduce waiting times but that would be perceived negatively by patients would be disregarded, while a proposed intervention that would reduce waiting times but that would be perceived as patient friendly would be considered.

Goals are used to provide direction for decision making. An organizational goal to increase market share in obstetrics influences management decisions when faced with prioritizing capital expenditures for remodeling patient care units in the hospital. An organizational goal of being the first-choice medical provider in the community may serve to motivate employees and other stakeholders. To promote an ideology or philosophy of care, such as the Planetree (2003) philosophy, a goal of "becoming a role model in patient-centered care" may be used. A goal to become a "center of excellence" for cardiovascular care may foster employee pride and loyalty, serve as a recruitment strategy for physicians and other clinical providers, and bring prestige within the community. A goal to be the "premier center for cancer research" can legitimize investment in research infrastructure at an academic medical center; successful research, in turn, will position the center well to acquire additional research funding

When used in conjunction with performance measurement, goals determine whether the data demonstrate favorable or unfavorable organizational performance. In the absence of either the goal or the measure, holding individuals accountable for improving performance or maintaining required competencies is difficult.

When managers realize how pervasively goals are used within the clinical and organizational settings, they may begin to appreciate the widespread impact that effective goal-setting skills may have on organizational performance. The importance of effective goals may be further appreciated when one realizes that all subsequent actions follow and are influenced by how the initial goal is set.

Relationship Between Goals and Results

The ability to set goals effectively is a requisite skill for managers at all levels of the organization. The following example of two hospitals facing a similar challenge illustrates how goals set by leadership influence subsequent actions and the results of those actions.

Hospital A and Hospital B both use a national vendor to measure and report their patient satisfaction. The reports show that both hospitals perform below the national average for hospitals of similar size and type. Senior leaders at each hospital decided to focus on improving customer service and patient satisfaction as an organizational priority. To address the problem of low patient satisfaction, the senior management team at Hospital A set the following goal: improve customer service.

To achieve this goal, Hospital A hired a customer service specialist and instituted mandatory customer service training for all employees. The nurse managers in the hospital were then faced with a dilemma. Their department education budgets were limited and their staff was already subject to mandatory education in areas such as infection control and fire safety. One more mandatory education would deplete the education dollars and eliminate the manager's resources for continuing education to maintain the staff's clinical competence.

When a goal offers little direction and is very vague, like Hospital A's goal, the result is often an approach to a type of problem solving called *repair service behavior,* where organizations or individuals solve a "problem" that they *know how* to solve whether or not it is the problem they *need* to solve (Dorner 1996). An example of repair service behavior is when a novice gardener responds to the problem of withering leaves on a new plant by watering the plant more instead of repotting and fertilizing, which are what the plant needs.

Hospital A knew how to create new positions and conduct training. However, it did not know how to identify the underlying cause of a widespread organizational problem. This example also illustrates how a poorly conceived goal (improve customer service) is likely to cause unintended consequences or even more problems in other areas of the organization. In this case, the mandatory customer service training took resources away from technical education and over time risked reducing the overall technical competency of the nursing staff.

Hospital B used a different approach to address the problem of low patient satisfaction. The senior management team at Hospital B set the following goals: (1) identify contributing factors to patient dissatisfaction, (2) prioritize the contributing factors, and (3) develop interventions to address the top-priority contributing factors. According to the hospital's satisfaction data, patients were most dissatisfied by lack of communication with nurses and with patient preparation for discharge. The organization conducted a root-cause analysis to learn the reasons that communication and discharge planning were not occurring effectively. The analysis revealed that, although staffing seemed adequate on a day-to-day basis, the hospital's reliance on temporary staff and traveling nurses had increased significantly over the past year. Although the temporary staff and traveling nurses were experienced in their technical duties, their lack of familiarity with the hospital's specific procedures and resources increasingly led to communication breakdowns both within and among departments. The organizational analysis highlighted this common problem for the departments responsible for patient registration, billing, and housekeeping as well as in the nursing, respiratory therapy, and pharmacy departments. On the basis of this information, senior leaders at Hospital B revised their goals as follows: (1) increase the proportion of staff who are permanent employees, (2) improve the discharge planning process, (2) reallocate resources spent on temporary staff to fund above improvements, and (4) monitor the impact of staffing and process improvements on patient satisfaction.

Because the source of the problem was not evident to Hospital B's administrators, they first set an intermediate goal of gaining a better understanding of why the problem was occurring. In so doing, they acknowledged the ways goals should be approached in complex systems such as healthcare organizations (Dorner 1996):

- When working with a complex, dynamic system, we must first develop at least a provisional picture of the partial goals we want to achieve; those partial goals will clarify what we need to do when.
- In complex situations, we must almost always avoid focusing on just one element and pursuing only one goal; instead, we must pursue several goals at once.

By stating its initial goal, Hospital B avoided an intervention that may not have solved the problem and was able to avoid the repair service behavior often associated with an unclear goal. Instead, Hospital B defined a clear, multiple-goal statement.

Approaches to Setting Goals

This section is not intended to teach managers how to do strategic planning. Rather, it provides managers with approaches that, once appropriate data are collected and preliminary problems are identified, they may use to assist them in setting effective goals for their own departments and organizations.

Use Intermediate Goals

Although vague, general, or unclear goals may lead to repair service behavior, general goals are useful to set the overall direction from which intermediate and specific goals can be established. In complex, dynamic systems such as healthcare organizations, partial or intermediate goals are often necessary to clarify what needs to be done. For example, a surgical services manager may use general goals to set the overall direction for his department. These goals may be to improve clinical outcomes, improve patient satisfaction, improve cost effectiveness, and integrate services across multiple sites. Each year, specific short-term goals or intermediate goals may also be established. The goal in Year 1 may be to implement a standard performance measurement system across all sites. The goal in Year 2 may be to increase the percentage of first surgical cases for the day that are started on time for each of the operating rooms in the service. The goal in Year 3 may be to implement standard preoperative testing protocols to eliminate unnecessary variation in preoperative tests (Kelly et al. 1997).

In this example, a general goal is used to communicate overall direction. Because the manager also understands the concept of partial goals, he is able to establish the first partial goal (measurement system) to help him understand how to prioritize subsequent annual improvement goals.

Define Implicit Goals

The surgical services manager in the example above also understands the concept of *implicit goals*—that is, a goal that may be intuitive but not necessarily purposefully addressed. For example, the manager knows that to achieve the desired level of performance, cultivating positive and collaborative relationships between physicians and administrators is essential. Although not explicitly defined in the manager's other performance goals, this implicit goal guides the approaches that the manager selected for designing the performance measurement system and for improving first-case start times. As a result of the manager's implicit goal of building relationships in years 1 and 2, implementing a clinical standard of care can be accomplished more smoothly in Year 3, which may not be possible without the benefit of improved working relationships between physicians and administrators.

Whenever possible, managers should try to identify implicit goals so they may be defined and communicated.

Reformulate Goals As Needed

Managers may find that setting goals is an iterative process; that is, as new information becomes available, managers must be willing to evaluate previous goals and reformulate goals as needed. For example, a nurse manager of a 30-bed, medical-surgical patient unit was faced with improving the overall performance of her unit. Because the unit was the major inpatient unit of a small community hospital, she was faced with a major overhaul rather than simply a single improvement. However, she also realized that the goal "overhaul performance" was too vague to identify specific interventions, expectations, and action plans for her staff.

She reformulated her original goal—"overhaul performance"—to more clearly establish the general direction of the performance improvement effort. Her new goals were as follows: (1) promote teamwork, (2) promote continuity of care, (3) meet or exceed local and national standards of care, (4) integrate performance improvement into the daily work environment, (5) promote staff satisfaction, and (6) improve cost effectiveness.

Set Multiple Goals

The nurse manager in the previous example demonstrated another important approach for setting effective goals. Because of the interrelationships among activities, processes, and other elements in healthcare organizations, managers will find that focusing on multiple interrelated goals is necessary. Although a single goal may be useful for a simple process improvement, a systems perspective suggests the need for setting multiple goals that may be carried out concurrently and/or sequentially to take into account the interrelationships within the system.

In this medical-surgical unit, the nurse manager assembled a team of charge nurses to work together intensively for a series of meetings to help determine how to meet the unit's goals. After several meetings directed toward understanding the hospital's history, operating requirements, and environmental challenges; analyzing current processes; and identifying causes of performance gaps, the team discussed its ideal vision for the unit. They described their ideal unit according to desired clinical outcomes, the nature of their relationships with patients and families, teamwork, and business requirements. This vision became the unit's long-term goal.

The members of the team realized that, to achieve this multifaceted vision, they must also focus on multiple interdependent interventions. They also realized that, although they were not able to implement multiple interventions all at once because of resource constraints, identifying, prioritizing, and establishing timelines for the multiple goals were important and served as the "roadmap" of their vision. The team found that some of the goals (e.g., establishing a staff communication book and bulletin board) could be implemented immediately without much effort. The team realized that some of the goals (e.g., improving the way in which daily census and productivity were tracked, reported, communicated, and managed) would take a month or so to implement and were identified as short-term goals. The team learned that some of the goals (e.g., clarifying care team roles, structure, and job descriptions) required more in-depth development and implementation considerations and were identified as medium-term goals.

The team realized and converted an implicit goal to an explicit one when it established the following long-term goal: enhance the personal accountability of all staff. Clear goals provided the direction, while a performance measurement system and a simple project tracking report enabled the manager, the team, and the unit staff to track their progress toward their goals and their progress toward becoming their ideal unit.

Types of Goal Statements

Along with understanding the various approaches used in setting effective goals, managers must purposefully craft a goal statement that will best help them succeed in a given situation. For example, a manager has just learned that the immunization rates for the patients in his large pediatric practice are below both the state and national averages. He is faced with the problem of substandard immunization rates. How does he now communicate improvement goals to the practice in ways that will enable him to utilize the approaches just described?

Some types of goal statements have been introduced through the examples presented earlier in the chapter. The different types of goals may be thought of as pairs of opposites: positive or negative, general or specific, clear or unclear, simple or multiple, and implicit or explicit (Dorner 1996). Table 7.1 provides a definition for each of these types and examples of how each may be used by the manager of the pediatric practice.

Conclusion

Effective goals precede effective performance. This chapter explores approaches that managers may use to improve their own goal-setting skills. Although no single correct or incorrect approach to setting a goal exists, managers should be aware of the advantages and pitfalls of each approach and the ways the goals are communicated. The exercise at the end of this chapter provides an opportunity to set goals in different ways, to critique the alternative goals, and to select the most appropriate and effective goal. Chapter 8 explores assumptions around another management norm: purpose. Often expressed as an organizational or departmental mission statement, a clear understanding and definition of purpose may be considered a high-leverage systemic structure.

Companion Reading

Dorner, D. 1996. *The Logic of Failure: Recognizing and Avoiding Error in Complex Situations,* 49–70. Reading, MA: Perseus Books.

TABLE 7.1
Examples of Goals

Definition	Type of Goal	Example
Working toward a desired condition versus making an undesirable condition go away	Positive	Achieve immunization rates that are in the top 10 percent statewide.
	Negative	Reduce the number of patients with incomplete immunizations.
Few criteria versus multiple criteria	General	Improve immunization rates.
	Specific	Ensure all infants in the practice receive the appropriate vaccinations at ages 1 month, 2 months, 4 months, 6 months, 12 months, 15 months, 18 months, and 24 months according to the Centers for Disease Control and Prevention Recommended Childhood Immunization Schedule.
Difficult to determine if the goal has been met versus precise criteria permitting the evaluation of whether the goal is being met	Unclear	Work with the office staff to improve pediatric care.
	Clear	Our clinic will select a team to enroll in the quality improvement course offered by the State Pediatric Association from April through September. The team will design and implement processes to improve the clinic's compliance with the Recommended Childhood Immunization Schedule. The team will measure overall immunization rates on a quarterly basis. Results will be reported at staff meetings.
Single goal versus series of sequential or concurrent goals that take into account relationships within the system	Simple	Give age-appropriate immunizations at each well-child appointment.
	Multiple	Track patient compliance with well-child exams. Notify and schedule patients who have missed well-child exams. Give age-appropriate immunizations during well-child exams.
Obvious versus hidden	Implicit	Improve immunization rates.
	Explicit	Improve the ability to identify, deliver, and monitor pediatric preventative care services, including age-appropriate immunizations.

Source: Dorner, D. 1996. *The Logic of Failure: Recognizing and Avoiding Error in Complex Situations.* Reading, MA: Perseus Books.

References

Bordley, W. C., P. A. Margolis, J. Stuart, C. Lannon, and L. Keyes. 2001. "Improving Preventive Service Delivery Through Office Systems." *Pediatrics* 108 (3): E41.

Dorner, D. 1996. *The Logic of Failure: Recognizing and Avoiding Error in Complex Situations.* Reading, MA: Perseus Books.

Jencks S. F., E. D. Huff, and T. Tuerdon. 2003. "Change in the Quality of Care Delivered to Medicare Beneficiaries, 1998–1999 to 2000–2001." *Journal of the American Medical Association* 289 (3): 305–12.

Kelly, D. L., S. L. Pestotnik, M. C. Coons, and J. W. Lelis. 1997. "Reengineering a Surgical Service Line: Focusing on Core Process Improvement." *American Journal of Medical Quality* 12 (2): 120–29.

Margolis, P. A., R. Stevens, W. C. Bordley, J. Stuart, C. Harlan, L. Keyes-Elstein, and S. Wisseh. 2001. "From Concept to Application: The Impact of a Community-wide Intervention to Improve the Delivery of Preventative Services to Children." *Pediatrics* 108 (3): E42.

Planetree. 2003. [Online information; retrieved 2/18/03]. http://www.plane-tree.org/.

Scott, W. R. 1998. *Organizations: Rational, Natural and Open Systems.* Upper Saddle River, NJ: Prentice Hall.

Exercise

Objective: To practice writing and critiquing different types of goal statements.

Instructions:

1. Read the following scenario.
2. State the problem in the scenario.
3. Review the different types of goal statements:
   a. Positive or negative
   b. General or specific
   c. Clear or unclear
   d. Simple or multiple
   e. Implicit or explicit
4. Choose two types of goal statements from the above list (e.g., a and b, a and d, c and e). Your goals for the scenario below should be stated using the two types of statements you selected; each type has two, so your goal should be stated four ways. List the pros and cons of each type of goal statement. Write your responses on a worksheet similar to the Goals Worksheet below.
5. Choose one of these goal statements as the goal to use in addressing the problem posed in the scenario. Describe your rationale for selecting this statement.

Scenario

You are the manager of an emergency department for a large acute care hospital. You have just reviewed your department's quality indicators, which are used to evaluate the quality of care for Medicare beneficiaries. You find that your hospital's performance on the indicators for care of patients with acute myocardial infarction is below the average performance of all hospitals in your state. You must improve performance in the following areas (Jencks, Huff, and Tuerdon 2003).

- Timeliness of administration of aspirin
- Prescribing aspirin at discharge
- Smoking cessation counseling

Your boss has asked you to present him with your improvement goals.

Goals Worksheet

Category	Goal Statement	Pros	Cons

PURPOSE

Objectives

- To explore the importance of purpose to quality management
- To gain an appreciation for the role of purpose in obtaining desired results
- To describe an approach for clarifying purpose
- To practice using the purpose principle

The quality department at Hospital A defined its mission as "Helping departments improve their quality indicators to meet regulatory requirements." The hospital had consistently met the JCAHO performance requirements and also demonstrated improvement on the clinical indicators for Medicare beneficiaries required by the Center for Medicare and Medicaid Services (CMS) (Jencks, Huff, and Tuerdon 2003). However, physicians at Hospital A consistently complained to the CEO about bottlenecks in scheduling x-ray examinations for their patients and delays in receiving results for just about any diagnostic test.

The quality department at Hospital B defined its mission as "Providing technical and consultative support to departments, managers, and teams to assist them in improving value to their customers." Hospital B also consistently met the JCAHO performance requirements and demonstrated improvement in the CMS clinical indicators. However, Hospital B also demonstrated improved cycle times in numerous clinical diagnostic processes, reduced its overall operational costs, and improved employee satisfaction and retention.

Organizations and departments often use a mission statement to define their identity. The mission statement states the reason the organization or department exists, the goals of the organization or department as a system, and the purpose of the organization or department. Although goals and purpose tend to overlap, these two concepts are treated separately in this book. The term *goal* refers to a desired end, while the term *purpose* refers to the reason for being. Like goals, purpose is also followed by subsequent actions influenced by the defined purpose. Often, after examining the purpose of an initiative, a manager may need to reevaluate, revise, and redefine the initial goals. In this way, purpose can be a tool to assist managers in reformulating partial or general goals to address the next level of specificity.

The quality department in Hospital A defined itself in terms of a single goal rather than purpose; the department was looking to attain specific results in accordance with defined performance indicators. Hospital A succeeded in achieving these results, but it was not successful in achieving an overall quality organization. In Hospital B, the quality department defined itself as a resource to others in the hospital to help improve the value of services provided. One of the quality department's goals may have been to improve care delivered to those patient populations addressed by the indicators. By improving the hospital's overall discharge process, for example, the department improved not only the ability to identify patients at risk for pneumonia and administer pneumococcal and influenza immunizations prior to discharge (required indicators) but also the overall quality of the patient and family's transition from the acute care setting to home, home care, or long-term care (Jencks, Huff, and Tuerdon 2003).

Managers should consciously and consistently question purpose at all levels of the organization—that is, the purpose of individual activities, jobs/roles, processes, departments, and the organization overall. A clear understanding of purpose guides managers in establishing direction for improvements, helps managers to know that they are working on the right problems, and increases the likelihood that quality efforts will achieve intended results. Without a clear understanding of purpose, managers run the risk of wasting time and resources working on the wrong problem or even improving something that should not exist in the first place.

This chapter explores the concept of purpose and its importance for managers. Approaches that managers may use to define, refine, and clarify purpose are also discussed.

The Importance of Purpose

In Chapter 1, Donabedian's causal relationship of quality-of-care measures was described as Structure ➡ Process ➡ Outcome. However, when designing or redesigning interventions to improve results, the sequence is conceptually reversed: a clear understanding of purpose should guide designing processes to support achieving that purpose, and the structure (how people are organized and roles are defined) should be guided by the requirements of the process. This sequence may be thought of as Purpose/Outcome ➡ Process ➡ Structure.

When using this conceptual sequence, understanding and clarifying purpose serves an important role in setting direction and ensuring that the right problem is being addressed. Discussions of purpose can also foster common ground and promote breakthrough ideas and solutions.

Setting Direction

A student's purpose or identity shapes his selection of classes. A student with an identity of musician may take music theory and instrument classes, while a medical student may choose anatomy and physiology classes. Similarly, the identity of an organization or units shapes its management choices of goals, priorities, resource allocation, and improvement targets.

A hospital-based laboratory performed tests for the inpatient and outpatient populations of the tertiary hospital in which it was located and for smaller hospitals and physicians' offices in the area. The manager and medical director, faced with the need to redesign the laboratory's operations, set a departmental goal to redesign the processes and the work area to improve efficiency and better meet customer needs; they organized a redesign team.

One of the first topics the redesign team discussed was the laboratory's purpose. Initially the team described the laboratory's purpose as providing customer service. For a hospital that had formally adopted a total quality philosophy several years previously, the team's focus on customer service indicated that they had integrated this total quality principle into their way of operating. However, to provide customer service was not a reason to exist; customer service was a part of what the laboratory provided but not its sole function. It was necessary to provide something other than customer service.

The redesign facilitator and the manager invited panels of internal customers to talk with the team about their own expectations and experiences as customers of this laboratory's service. The common theme heard from each customer, whether a nurse in the emergency room or a doctor's office, was that they depended on the information that the laboratory gave them to make patient care decisions. In their efforts to provide quality service, the laboratory had lost sight of the reason it existed: to provide information. The team realized that quality service was a desired characteristic in how they delivered the information.

As the team continued to discuss the laboratory's purpose, the team also realized that they provided customers with three distinct types of information. The first type of information was clinical patient data in the form of test results. Within this "product line" were numerous types of results from many types of specimens, from blood for analyzing cholesterol levels to tissue for analyzing a cancerous tumor. Over the years, however, the laboratory's role had evolved in response to managed care, new technology, and published research on clinical treatments and interventions. As a result, the laboratory found itself providing its customers with two additional "product lines": (1) information in the form of technical expertise to other providers about how to use and interpret the new tests as they became available and (2) information related to the technical and regulatory requirements as more tests moved away from the laboratory to point-of-care techniques carried out by nurses or physicians.

Clarifying its purpose became an empowering realization for the laboratory staff. Each of the three product lines of information was necessary to provide laboratory services to all of its customers; however, only one—

clinical laboratory results—was a potential source of measurable revenue or expense for this department; the other two product lines were solely a source of expense for the department. Equipped with a clear definition of purpose and arguing with a systems point of view, the laboratory manager and medical director were able to negotiate budgetary expectations with their administrator. They were able to articulate that the laboratory may be incurring expenses that ultimately benefited the quality of patient care in other departments and/or reduced the cost of the patient's total hospital experience. The budget discussions changed from focusing exclusively on reducing laboratory expenses to including how to measure and preserve the laboratory's essential role in providing overall quality of laboratory services to all patients within its service domain, not simply for work carried out within the boundaries of the laboratory's walls (Kelly 1998).

Addressing the Right Problem

The manager in an ambulatory surgery unit was faced with the problem of frequent patient delays that led to patient complaints and higher costs as a result of excessive length of stay. The manager assembled a team to address the goal of redesigning patient flow to improve clinical outcomes, patient satisfaction, and cost effectiveness (Kelly et al. 1997).

In one of the first redesign meetings, the facilitator asked the team to identify the major phases of care comprising the entire process of care for a patient experiencing ambulatory surgery. The team identified five phases that an ambulatory surgery patient receives: (1) the prehospital phase—that is, care occurring somewhere other than in the ambulatory surgery unit; (2) the preoperative phase—that is, care occurring in the ambulatory surgery unit before the patient goes to the operating room; (3) the intraoperative phase—that is, the actual operation taking place in the operating room; (4) the postoperative phase—that is, care supporting patient recovery and taking place in the recovery room or the ambulatory surgery unit; and (5) the posthospitalization phase—that is, care occurring after the patient is discharged from the ambulatory surgery unit; this may include a follow-up phone call by a nurse or follow-up care in the physician's office.

The facilitator then asked the team to select an area that, if improved, could have the most impact on improving patient flow and reducing delays. The team chose the prehospital phase because this process was "upstream" to all of the others. If delays or breakdowns occurred during this phase of care, the rest of the process would also be delayed.

Next, the facilitator led a discussion about the purpose of the prehospital phase of care. Immediately the team replied, "To prepare the patient for surgery; to make sure the patient is ready." As the purpose discussion continued, the team had a breakthrough when they realized that, although the prehospital phase of care helped to prepare the patient, its primary purpose was to prepare the hospital to receive and care for the patient in the most effective and efficient manner. If this occurred, the patient was more likely to progress through the other phases of care without unnecessary delays or surprises. This realization of purpose, along with the understanding of the interconnectedness of operational and clinical processes (see the "Three Core Process Model" section in Chapter 5), played an important role in redesigning the patient flow process.

Other efforts within the organization to redesign the patient pre-registration process achieved just that—a reengineered preregistration process. An understanding of the purpose of the prehospital phase of care led the surgery team to look at preregistration in a different way. The team identified an entire package of information required prior to the patient's admission that helped to prepare the care providers and the facility to most efficiently provide the service of outpatient surgery. This package not only included registration information (e.g., patient demographics, insurance data) but also patient education materials, clinical preparation of the patient (e.g., laboratory results, special orders, patient history), surgery schedul-ing, and information about the surgical procedure so that any special equip-ment or supplies could be arranged for in advance. The preadmission infor-mation-gathering process was then designed to promote assembling this package of information during a patient encounter at the physician's office and making sure that the information package had arrived at the hospital in advance of the patient's admission. A phone call to the patient the day before surgery confirmed last-minute details and provided the opportunity to answer any additional patient questions. In this way, the facility and care providers were better prepared to receive the patient, provide individual-ized care, anticipate and prevent delays or cancellations as a result of mis-communication or lack of information, and decrease the preoperative length of stay (Kelly et al. 1997).

Fostering Common Ground

Without a clear understanding of what has to be accomplished, discussions on alternative solutions to a problem may often lead to impasses. Selecting one approach over another is hindered because people often bring to the discussion their own intense ownership of a particular solution, interven-tion, or idea. Discussing purpose can be a less-threatening way to begin a discussion about a problem. Rather than highlighting differences among possible options and inviting comments on their perceived merit or short-comings, discussing purpose helps to create a common ground from which to focus people with divergent opinions and views.

Information systems are used in healthcare organizations for a vari-ety of purposes: storing, retrieving, and streamlining and automating access to data. Many information systems began as accounting systems. As more clinical applications are being developed and demands for electronic med-ical records and computerized physician order entry increase, questioning the purpose of these systems is important to ensure that the purpose, applications, uses, and outcomes are all aligned.

The clinical epidemiology and medical informatics team at LDS Hospital in Salt Lake City, Utah, has used computerized systems to improve patient care for more than 20 years. In 1998, an article appeared in the *New England Journal of Medicine* that described the evaluation of LDS Hospital's computer-assisted management program for antibiotics and other anti-infective agents (Evans et al. 1998). (For more information on the details of the technology, see the reference list at the end of this chapter.) Managers must understand how the LDS Hospital's team defined the purpose of clinical information systems: "The project was designed to augment physicians' judgment, not to replace it. The computer was simply a tool that offered data on individual patients, decision logic, and prescribing information to physicians in a useful and non-threatening way" (Garibaldi 1998).

The purpose of the clinical information system was to support decision making, and this in turn fostered cooperation between information systems and the clinicians. Too often the purposes of a clinical information system are to control behavior rather than to support it, to reduce practitioner autonomy rather than enhance it, and to fulfill administrator requirements rather than patient and clinician requirements. These purposes foster adversarial rather than cooperative relationships. The clear description of the purpose can create common ground for the team and practitioners, contribute to focusing on a common goal, and enlist practitioner buy-in to successfully use innovative technology to improve patient outcomes.

Promoting Breakthrough Ideas and Solutions

In Chapter 3, the process tool called lead-time analysis was introduced. The user of this tool physically walks through the steps of a process, notes the time it takes to complete a process step, measures the distance between steps, and analyzes the steps to determine if the process step contributes value to the overall process.

By using lead-time analysis, one team member of the laboratory redesign effort described earlier discovered the cumbersome and time-consuming process required for a test-result report to travel from the laboratory to the physician's office across the street. A clear understanding of the laboratory's purpose (to provide information) helped the team to ask the right questions before trying to improve this process. Previously the team may have asked, "How can we improve the process of delivering the results via the mail?" The team's understanding of purpose caused them to instead ask, "How can we get the information to the physician's office in the most timely manner?" By asking the improvement question this way, the team began to identify alternatives to mail and ultimately installed a fax server into the laboratory information system. The fax server enabled the laboratory to send test results directly to a physician's office's fax machine to improve the timeliness with which customers received laboratory results while at the same time improving customer satisfaction (Kelly 1998).

This example may sound very simple; however, it also demonstrates the value of understanding purpose. Had the laboratory designed an intervention on the basis of its original purpose, the department may have improved the mail process or added staff to the customer service team. Instead, when it focused on its real purpose, the department was able to design a much more effective solution.

The "Purpose Principle"

The examples in this chapter illustrate that, as our healthcare systems grow in complexity, forgetting to periodically evaluate our purpose becomes easy. Managers must develop the habit of asking themselves, "What are we really trying to achieve? On the basis of changes in the environment, technology, or customer requirements, what is our purpose? Does our current method of operating serve that purpose, or are there more effective alternatives?" When the purpose is clear, new solutions usually become clear as well.

The *purpose principle* comes from the concept of breakthrough thinking (Nadler and Hibino 1994), an approach to problem solving developed from studying effective leaders and problem solvers from various industries and disciplines. Nadler and Hibino (1994) found that "when confronted with a problem, successful people tend to question why they should spend their time and effort solving the problem at all" and that effective problem solvers "always placed every problem into a larger context . . . to understand the relationship between what effective action on the problem was *supposed* to achieve and the purposes of the larger setting of which the original problem was a part." By questioning purpose and enlarging the boundaries from which they examined the problem, effective problem solvers were able to purposely and systematically choose the right problem and the best solution.

When examined from a systems thinking perspective, using the purpose principle promotes double-loop learning by challenging assumptions about the nature of a problem. By encouraging the viewing of the problem and solution from the larger context of the entire system, the purpose principle also promotes an understanding of the connections between the problem at hand and other elements or components of the system.

From Concept to Practice

A series of questions can help managers to examine and clarify purpose. The first question should be, "What am I trying to accomplish," or "what is this process, intervention, or department designed to accomplish?" By asking this question first, a discussion of purpose and accompanying mental models regarding the problem and solution may be brought out into the open.

The next question involves expanding the purpose. Expanding the purpose is not meant to reduce the problem to a lesser problem but to identify and understand how the problem is related to the overall context in which it exists. Think of an onion. The effort of expanding the purpose is actually like starting from the inside of an onion and adding on the layers to construct a whole onion rather than peeling the onion, as this is typically the case when the onion metaphor is used. When purpose is identified, questions like, "And we do that because?" follow. In this way, the larger purposes may be identified—more layers are added to the onion. When the original purpose has been expanded several times, then another question should be asked: "What larger purpose might eliminate the need to achieve this smaller purpose?" (Nadler and Hibino 1994). Population approaches used in public health often provide solutions in this way. Rather than finding better ways to treat diseases caused by water-borne organisms, early public health practitioners devised ways to eliminate the organisms from drinking water. Similarly, vaccinations like the polio vaccine are solutions to a larger purpose (preventing the disease) rather than a smaller purpose (treating the disease).

By questioning, identifying, and documenting different purposes, the manager or team may then select the level of purpose most appropriate to solve, which is the purpose that enables them to solve the right problem and that is within their means (e.g., resources, scope of authority). At first the questions may be difficult to answer and may appear to be redundant. However, like anything new, with practice the ability to answer the questions will improve, and the repetition will encourage a deeper level of thinking about the problem.

Here is an example of how one may approach a problem using the purpose principle and answering the above questions. A manager at a local community center is faced with the problem of inconsistent collection of fees for wellness classes sponsored by the center. Community center members have unlimited use of the swimming pool and exercise equipment. The center also offers members a variety of wellness classes for a small fee, which is intended to cover the cost of the instructors and materials. Some classes are taught at the center by the center's staff, but some classes are taught by instructors employed by local healthcare providers. For example, a class on low-fat menus may be sponsored by the wellness program but taught at the local hospital by the hospital's dietitian. Collecting fees for the classes offered on site is not a problem because class participants are required to check in at the reception desk. However, for those classes taking place off-site, the collection rate is barely 50 percent. The center has also received numerous complaints from course instructors that either too many or not enough participants showed up for a particular class.

The manager may ask himself the following questions:

- What am I trying to accomplish?
  To collect fees from class enrollees
- Have I expanded the purposes of addressing the problem? I collect fees from class enrollees because . . . ?
  To increase revenue, we need to have accurate record keeping, including who has registered, who has attended, and who has paid for the class. We also have to make sure the fees we charge cover the costs of the class instructors and materials.
- The purpose of increasing revenues, having accurate record keeping, and covering the costs of instructors and material is to . . . ?
  To cover our own expenses if we want to continue to offer a wide variety of classes taught by quality instructors
- The purpose of covering our expenses is to . . . ?
  To remain financially sound and to continue to provide wellness services for the community
- My customers' purposes are to . . . ?
  The purposes of the instructors are to offer their classes with minimal logistics and administrative hassles (e.g., compensation, paperwork) and to be prepared for their classes. The purposes of the members are to stay healthy and to have a place for social interaction.
- What larger purpose may eliminate the need to achieve this smaller purpose altogether?
  If I had a grant or if community partners donated money, time, or staff, we would not have to worry about charging members and collecting fees.
- What is the right problem for me to be working on?
  To improve the logistics and administrative processes to provide a low-hassle teaching environment for our instructors and low-hassle classes for our members.

Although the initial focus for this manager was to collect more money, after answering this series of questions, he realized that the center had not explicitly defined or communicated the roles and expectations of the community center staff, the class participants, or the class instructors for an off-site offering. One expectation was about how and when payment should be collected. As a result, the manager changed his focus from collecting money to defining and communicating expectations. He then identified a variety of interventions to help with this new purpose, including changing the content of class brochures and posters, holding an orientation meeting with off-site instructors, setting registration deadlines so a final participant roster can be faxed to instructors at least 24 hours in advance, and assigning a community center staff member as a liaison to assist the instructor with logistics and fee collection. The manager also began to think about how he could engage financial support from local providers to help defray some of the costs.

Conclusion

This chapter introduces the concept and role of purpose in quality management. The companion reading section below provides a detailed description of the purpose principle and a more in-depth explanation of how managers may approach it. The exercise at the end of this chapter has been designed to provide the opportunity to practice the purpose principle and to become more acquainted with how to apply this concept to a healthcare problem. Chapter 9 discusses the role of measurement in quality management and offers measurement lessons from a systems thinking perspective.

Companion Reading

Nadler, G., and S. Hibino. 1994. *Breakthrough Thinking: The Seven Principles of Creative Problem Solving,* 17–37, 127–59. Rocklin, CA: Prima Publishing.

References

Evans, R. S., S. L. Pestotnik, D. C. Classen, T. P. Clemmer, L. K. Weaver, J. F. Orme, J. F. Lloyd, and J. P. Burke. 1998. "A Computer-Assisted Management Program for Antibiotics and Other Antiinfective Agents." *New England Journal of Medicine* 338 (4): 232–38.

Garibaldi, R. A. 1998. "Computers and the Quality of Care—A Clinician's Perspective." *New England Journal of Medicine* 338 (4): 259–60.

Jencks S. F., E. D. Huff, and T. Tuerdon. 2003. "Change in the Quality of Care Delivered to Medicare Beneficiaries, 1998–1999 to 2000–2001." *Journal of the American Medical Association* 289 (3): 305–12.

Kelly, D. L. 1998. "Reframing Beliefs About Work and Change Processes in Redesigning Laboratory Services." *Joint Commission Journal on Quality Improvement* 24 (9): 154–67.

Kelly, D. L., S. L. Pestotnik, M. C. Coons, and J. W. Lelis. 1997. "Reengineering a Surgical Service Line: Focusing on Core Process Improvement." *American Journal of Medical Quality* 12 (2): 120–29.

Nadler, G., and S. Hibino. 1994. *Breakthrough Thinking: The Seven Principles of Creative Problem Solving.* Rocklin, CA: Prima Publishing.

Exercise

Objective: To practice using the purpose principle

Instructions:

Read the following scenario. Write your responses to the questions afterward.

Scenario

You are the office manager for a large obstetrics and gynecology practice that is part of a larger multispecialty clinic. The clinic administration has implemented a new performance management system. When you are given the first "clinic report card," the data show that, for obstetrical patients, your practice has performed very well in the area of pregnancy-associated complications. However, the practice has performed poorly in the areas of patient satisfaction. In particular, patients are not satisfied with their level of involvement in their own care and their preparation for labor, delivery, breastfeeding, and care of their newborns.

You know your staff are committed to quality patient care and are very hard workers. Out of curiosity, you ask one of the obstetricians, "What is the purpose of prenatal care and the prenatal office visits?" The physician replies, "To identify signs of problems with the mother or the fetus and to intervene early to prevent them from getting worse." You ask the physician what kinds of problems may potentially occur, to which she replies, "Things like toxemia in the mother or growth retardation in the fetus." You identify your problem as patient dissatisfaction with prenatal care. You identify the process as prenatal care. You identify the purpose of the prenatal visits as described by the physician: early identification and intervention of problems with the mother and the fetus or baby.

Practice the purpose principle by asking yourself the following questions:

1. What am I trying to accomplish?
2. Have I expanded the purposes of addressing this problem? The purpose of (response to #1) is to . . . ?
3. Have I further expanded the purpose? The purpose of (response to #2) is to . . . ?
4. Have I further expanded the purpose? The purpose of (response to #3) is to . . . ?
5. For physicians, the purpose of prenatal care is . . . ?
6. For patients, the purpose of prenatal care is . . . ?
7. For the insurance companies, the purpose of prenatal care is . . . ?
8. What larger purpose may eliminate the need to achieve this smaller purpose altogether?
9. What is the right purpose for me to be working on? Describe how this purpose differs or does not differ from my original purpose.

PERFORMANCE MEASUREMENT

Objectives

- To describe the essential role of measurement in quality management
- To presents systems lessons on using performance measurement
- To introduce concepts related to process variation
- To practice constructing and interpreting statistical process control charts

B aseball scores, the weather report, interest rates, even grass height satisfy our need for measurement. We are accustomed to using data to make decisions and monitor our personal interests, whether we are following the progress of our favorite sports team, determining how to dress, deciding to buy a house, or knowing when to mow the lawn.

Individuals use data to guide their own healthcare activities. A child's hot forehead alerts a mother to the possibility of a fever. A grandmother with diabetes measures her daily blood sugar level to regulate her insulin dosage. People exercise 20 minutes a day, three times a week to remain fit. Care providers use data to diagnose, treat, and monitor clinical conditions and the effectiveness of interventions. Blood tests, x-rays, and vital signs all provide information to enhance the care provider's effectiveness. In each of these examples, data add value to the process. Data give us information about something we are interested in, help us to choose among various options, alert us when something needs to be done, and define the boundaries of an activity.

When we follow our favorite sports team during the course of the season, we are looking at data over time for trends and progress. When we check to see what place the team is in relation to the other teams in the same division, we are comparing data points. When we realize our lawn is high compared with the neighbors', we are using a benchmark to signal that we need to mow the grass. If we check the weather report for the barometric pressure or chance of rain, we are using formal measures. When we use our hand to check a forehead for fever, we are measuring informally.

Healthcare managers often forget these measurement lessons from other parts of life. In healthcare organizations, measurement may occur by default—that is, we measure what we can measure. Measurement may occur because it is required by regulatory agencies such as JCAHO, and rules from other industries may dictate measurement systems such as monthly, quarterly, or annual financial statements. While immersed in data and reporting, healthcare managers face the risk of being "data rich and information poor" about how their unit, department, or organization is actually performing.

This chapter discusses measurement as the foundation for organizational effectiveness, lists several systems lessons for using measurement in improving and managing performance, and reviews process variation that affects quality.

The Foundation for Organizational Effectiveness

Although managers may successfully report the performance indicators required by internal and external stakeholders, they may still not be successfully managing their organizations. Managers must recognize the difference between reporting indicators and measuring performance. According to the Baldrige National Quality Program (2003), "measurement and analysis are critical to the effective management of your organization and to a fact-based system for improving health care and operational performance" and "serve as a foundation for the performance management system." In other words, measurement is essential to managing and improving organizational performance and results. Therefore, managers must see performance—not simply performance indicators—as the end result of their efforts.

The thought of designing, implementing, and using performance measures may seem overwhelming at first to a healthcare manager. However, when performance measurement is viewed as a process, steps may be taken to initiate, carry out, and continually improve the process. Figure 9.1 describes a continuum that a manager or organization may use to determine the maturity of a performance measurement system. As shown in Figure 9.1, those embarking on new or early efforts are on the far left of the continuum and may have few or no reported results. Those who are experienced in their efforts are shown on the far right and are characterized by not only what and how performance is reported but also by results that demonstrate improvement over time and show leadership within their industries (Baldrige National Quality Program 2003).

In recent years, availability and access to comparative data in healthcare has greatly improved. Table 9.1 provides several sources that managers may use in comparing their organizations' performance to that of other organizations.

Lessons for Healthcare Managers

Managers must purposefully select indicators and design a measurement system that is linked to and aligned with their organizations' goals, business strategy, and customer and stakeholder requirements. The manager should also consider the lessons in this section when selecting and using indicators in a performance measurement system.

FIGURE 9.1

The Continuum of Maturity in Performance Management

There are no results or poor results in areas reported

There are some improvements and/or early good performance levels in a few areas

Results are not reported for many to most areas of importance to your key organizational requirements

Improvements and/or good performance levels are reported in many areas of importance to your key organizational requirements

Early stages of developing trends and obtaining comparative information are evident

Results are reported for many to most areas of importance to your key organizational requirements

Improvement trends and/or good performance levels are reported for most areas of importance to your key organizational requirements

No pattern of adverse trends and no poor performance levels are evident in areas of importance to your key organizational requirements

Some trends and/or current performance levels-evaluated against relevant comparisons and/or benchmarks-show areas of strength and/or good to very good relative performance levels

Organizational performance results address most key customer, market, and process requirements

Beginning Efforts ⟶ **Mature Efforts**

Source: Adapted from National Institute of Standards and Technology. 2003. "Baldrige National Quality Program Health Care Criteria for Performance Excellence." Gaithersburg, MD: National Institute of Standards and Technology.

TABLE 9.1
Sources of
Comparative
Data for
Healthcare
Managers

Patient Satisfaction

- Picker Survey (National Research Corporation)

  http://www.patient experiencestandard.org
  http://www.nationalresearch.com/
- Press Ganey Associates   http://www.pressganey.com/
- The Gallup Organization   http://www.gallup.com/

Practice Patterns

- Leatherman, S., and D. McCarthy. 2002. *Quality of Healthcare in the United States: A Chartbook*. New York: The Commonwealth Fund.
- The Center for the Evaluative Clinical Sciences, Dartmouth Medical School. 1996. *The Dartmouth Atlas of Healthcare*. Chicago: The American Hospital Publishing Company.

Health Plans

- National Committee for Quality Assurance (NCQA) HEDIS measures

  http://www.ncqa.org/index.htm

Clinical Indicators

- Joint Commission on Accreditation of Healthcare Organizations (JCAHO) ORYX measures

  http://www.jcaho.org/pms/index.htm
- Centers for Medicare and Medicaid (CMS) Medicare Clinical Indicators

  http://www.cms.gov/qio/2.asp

Population Measures

- State and local health departments
- Centers for Disease Control and Prevention National Center for Health Statistics

  http://www.cdc.gov/nchs/

Choose a Balanced Set of Measures

Managers should use a varied and balanced set of measures or indicators to ensure that one area of performance is not unintentionally excelling at the expense of another.

An approach called the *balanced scorecard* has been described in business literature (Kaplan and Norton 1992, 1993, 1996; *Harvard*

Management Update) and in healthcare literature (Aidemark 2001; Chow et al. 1998; Inamdar, Kaplan, and Bower 2002; Inamdar et al. 2000; Jason 2001; Zelman et al. 1999). The balanced scorecard is a "set of measures that gives top managers a fast but comprehensive view of the business" (Kaplan and Norton 1992). Data are reported in specific categories that represent four perspectives of the organization's performance: (1) the customer perspective, (2) the internal perspective, (3) the innovation and learning perspective, and (4) the financial perspective (Kaplan and Norton 1992).

The *clinical value compass* may be thought of as a balanced scorecard for evaluating outcomes of a clinical process. The four categories that it measures (the points of the compass) are functional status and well-being, satisfaction against need, costs, and clinical status (Nelson et al. 1996). These four points may be used to measure, evaluate, and improve the effectiveness of a clinical process, and they may also serve as a guide for managers when selecting metrics to measure, evaluate, and improve the performance of their departments or organizations (Kelly et al. 1997).

When choosing performance indicators, managers must balance the categories (i.e., using the balanced scorecard or clinical value compass approaches) and the types of measures. The three types of medical quality indicators are structure measures, process measures, and outcome measures. Tools, resources, characteristics of providers, settings, and organizations are considered *structure measures* (Donabedian 1980); examples of these types of measures are the number of hospital beds, the number of physicians on staff, and the age of the radiology equipment. Activities that occur between patients and providers—what is done to the patient—are considered *process measures* (Brook, Kamberg, and McGlynn 1996; Fitzgerald, Moore, and Dittus 1988). Preventative care activities such as mammography, immunization, and patients receiving prenatal care during the first trimester are examples of process measures. Changes in clinical status—what happens to the patient—are considered *outcome measures* (Brook, Kamberg, and McGlynn 1996; Donabedian 1980). The number of enrolled women who get a mammogram is a process measure, while the number of women who die from breast cancer is an outcome measure.

These three types of measures should also be considered when defining and selecting operational and management indicators. The proportion of new graduates to experienced staff is a structure measure, the number of staff who attended an in-service education class is a process measure, and the number of patient complaints is an outcome measure.

Translate Data into Information

Measures should reflect the performance of the entity that is being managed; therefore, a large hospital may have several levels and scopes of measurement. The CEO may review hospitalwide measures, a service line manager may focus on measures for a specific group of departments or patients, a department manager may focus on measures for his or her department, and a shift supervisor may focus on measures for a particular shift. All levels of performance indicators should reflect the common direction and priorities defined by the organization's mission, vision, and business strategy. A comprehensive performance measurement system should also ensure coordination among levels to minimize the duplication of collecting, reporting, and analyzing efforts.

Note that, as data are aggregated, some performance information may become buried in the data and that important opportunities for evaluation and improvement may be missed. For example, throughout the 1990s, hospital administrators used a common strategy of changing the ratio of professional staff and assistant personnel to reduce the average hourly wage expenses and in turn the overall personnel costs. Administrators of a large tertiary hospital that used this staffing strategy tracked staff turnover rates as one of the hospital's performance indicators. In 1995, turnover for the nursing department was at 25 percent, which was considered by the administrators to be reasonable given the local employment and economic environments. However, the nurse managers and nurses consistently voiced their concerns about understaffing and turnover.

When different levels of the organization are telling different stories about the operating environment, unbundling or disaggregating the indicators can be a useful strategy to evaluate the appropriateness of performance measures. When the nursing department's turnover data were examined more closely, all personnel in the department were found to be included in the calculations of turnover. The aggregate turnover figures reflected the combined turnover of registered nurses, licensed practical nurses, certified nurse assistants, and unit secretaries. Although the departmental turnover was 25 percent, the registered nurse turnover was 15 percent and the certified nursing assistant turnover was 43 percent. The potential salary savings for the lower-paid certified nursing assistants was essentially neutralized by the cost of recruiting, hiring, and training the constantly changing stream of these assistants.

In addition, while studying the departmental turnover data, the human resources department realized that internal staff transfers were not included in the turnover calculations and only included terminations. When staff movement within the organization was also taken into account, the turnover figures significantly underestimated the impact of staff changes on both the nursing managers and the frontline nursing staffs. Once these flaws in the performance indicators were identified, the human resources department redesigned its performance indicators and reporting mechanisms to account for changing activity at the unit level in addition to aggregate turnover at the departmental or organizational level.

Evaluate Results and Ongoing Results

A manager may evaluate both the performance of a specific intervention and ongoing performance. The Shewhart Cycle (see Chapter 3) provides a framework for collecting and reviewing data for a specific improvement intervention. This type of evaluation is illustrated in an improvement effort conducted by a group of anesthesiologists. When a new protocol for pre-operative laboratory test requirements was implemented, the follow-up measurement was important to evaluate both the degree to which the protocol was being followed and the impact of the new protocol on test use. One year later, evaluation data showed that unnecessary blood tests on patients undergoing tonsillectomy/adenoidectomy surgery declined by 51 percent and that unnecessary blood tests on patients undergoing arthroscopic knee surgery declined by 38 percent (Kelly et al. 1997).

For ongoing operations, the Shewhart Cycle suggests that managers should review performance indicators on a regular basis; plan appropriate interventions, if needed; implement appropriate solutions; and then continue to regularly review performance indicators. Some indicators, such as patient census, may be reported daily, weekly, monthly, quarterly, and annually. The reporting interval for a specific indicator will depend on customer and stakeholder requirements, intended uses, and organizational capabilities and resources. For example, measures used for ongoing operations in a multisite surgical services division included patient volumes, cost, patient satisfaction, clinical outcomes, and indicators related to specific service line improvement goals for that year. At monthly manager meetings, in addition to a more detailed monthly financial report, each manager received two performance reports: a service line performance report and a site-specific performance report. During these meetings, the managers reviewed, analyzed, and discussed the data; identified both good performance trends and areas of concern; and explored potential solutions and interventions. The check/study, act, and plan stages of the Shewhart cycle took place in a collaborative fashion among the unit managers in the service line. In the time between the monthly meetings, the managers were responsible for the "do" stage of the cycle, if required. By doing this, the management team used a monthly Shewhart Cycle to incorporate the performance measures into the overall performance management system (Kelly et al. 1997).

Understand the Relationship Between System and Component Measures

Historically, functional management structures in healthcare organizations have promoted component measures. It is not uncommon for hospitals to measure department-specific costs per unit of service. The laboratory may measure costs per test, while the pharmacy may measure costs per prescription. Because patients receive care from multiple departments within the hospital or along the continuum of care, managers must recognize and balance component and system costs from the organization's point of view and the patient's point of view.

For example, from the organization's point of view, the cost of an expensive drug from the pharmacy is acceptable if the drug allows the patient's overall length of stay to be reduced. Alternatively, the hospital can reduce the cost of an episode of care by cutting its discharge planner positions and thereby reducing its personnel expense. From the patient's point of view, however, an unnecessary readmission to the hospital can be avoided if the patient receives adequate home care instructions from a discharge planner. Although the hospital may be able to save money on a single episode of care, the overall cost of care to the healthcare system will increase because of a readmission that could have been avoided if adequate discharge preparation was offered the first time.

Managers, especially at higher levels in the organization, must be conscious of the interrelationships between system and component measures as they are establishing departmental and organizational performance direction and goals. When measures are viewed from a systems perspective, some components of the system may be intentionally suboptimized to optimize performance of the entire system. Likewise, some components of the system may be unintentionally optimized at the expense of the performance of the entire system.

Consider the redesign of an ambulatory surgery unit as an example. The redesign revealed that, as the clinical protocol for preoperative laboratory tests was revised to eliminate unnecessary tests (Kelly et al. 1997), the remaining blood tests could be conducted using point-of-care testing instruments. This new process eliminated the need for specimens to be transported to the hospital laboratory to be analyzed and for the results to be communicated back to the unit. The streamlined process cut 30 to 45 minutes from the preoperative length of stay. If the decision to go with the point-of-care testing was made based solely on cost per test, the new process would not have been implemented; the point-of-care cost per test was about five times greater than when the procedure was done in the laboratory. However, the savings and efficiencies gained by reducing unnecessary preoperative length of stay far outweighed the few dollars' difference in the cost per laboratory test.

Balancing system and component measures when allocating departmental resources and monitoring the impact of improvement efforts requires collaboration, negotiation, and awareness of the larger picture. The example in Chapter 8 concerning the laboratory's purpose also shows the need for negotiation and intentionally addressing the issue of system and component measures. The hospital in which the laboratory operated used the practice of benchmarking to establish performance targets for its managers. This laboratory demonstrated a higher cost per test than the benchmark data. The definition of purpose, however, enabled the manager to describe to his administrator that, although the higher cost per test reflected the expense incurred by the lab for consulting with other units, the benefit of savings was realized by other units or the hospital overall. The administrator and manager could then set more appropriate performance targets that took into account the differences between the practice of this laboratory and the practices that generated the benchmarking data.

Balancing system and component measures becomes more of a challenge when addressing continuum-of-care issues. Managers may include measures of unintended consequences in their overall performance measures to better understand the impact of their own interventions on others. In Chapter 4, an example was introduced that illustrated dynamic complexity in healthcare systems. Let us look at this same example from a measurement perspective. Following is a review of the example. The advent of prospective payment systems in the 1980s drove many hospitals to cut costs by reducing length of stay. An unintended consequence of this practice was that it shifted the monetary, functional, and quality-of-life costs to a downstream service or unit in the continuum of care or to the patients themselves. Table 4.1 illustrates the unintended consequences of reducing hospital length of stay for patients who received total hip arthroplasty.

Managers, financial officers, chief executive officers, and policymakers must all be aware of how decisions made and implemented within their domain of responsibility affect other parts of the healthcare system, both positively and negatively. They should ask themselves the following questions:

• Who is affected by this intervention?
• Who affects this intervention?
• What are possible unintended consequences of this intervention?
• Am I measuring the right thing?
• Have I included a measure of unintended consequences in my evaluation of the intervention?
• Am I unintentionally shifting costs to another component of the healthcare system?

Process Variation

Anyone who depends on public transportation has firsthand experience with process variation. If you have missed a bus because the driver was ahead of schedule or if you have been late for work because the driver was behind schedule, you have experienced the inconvenience and cost of variation in a process.

In Chapter 1, the goals of quality improvement were described as improving average performance and reducing the variation from the average to ensure more consistent results each time the process is carried out.

These goals were illustrated with a frequency distribution in Figure 1.3. A statistical process control chart is a valuable tool that can assist managers in monitoring, identifying, explaining, and managing variation in performance data. An in-depth explanation of statistical process control charts is beyond the scope of this book. However, in this section we present an overview of the basic concepts that can assist a manager in understanding and using statistical process control charts.

Statistical Process Control Charts

A *statistical process control chart* is a way of displaying performance data to enhance a manager's ability to identify variation in performance. Think of a process that is performed many times. The results are plotted on a frequency distribution, with the x-axis representing the value observed and the y-axis representing the number of times that value is observed. If the process is measured many times, a normal distribution—a bell curve—begins to take shape. Several measures may be derived from this normal distribution, including a measure of central tendency, such as a mean or average, and a measure of spread or distance from the mean, such as a standard deviation.

The total range of performance of the process is essentially captured by those values bounded by the mean plus three standard deviations above and below the mean. The boundaries established by the mean plus or minus two standard deviations will capture the process approximately 95 percent of the time (see Figure 9.2). When the frequency distribution is turned on its side, with the x-axis showing increments of time (e.g., day, month, quarter) and the y-axis showing the performance for that time period, the manager has constructed a control chart (see Figure 9.3). In this way, the manager may track and compare performance over time.

Key Concepts

A manager may get started using control charts with a few underlying concepts. First, "the Voice of the Customer defines what you want from a system" (Wheeler 2000). This phrase is another way of stating the concepts introduced in Chapter 2 of customer expectations and of patient and other stakeholder requirements. If an organization desires to be customer- or patient-focused, its processes must be rooted in the requirements of its patients, customers, and other stakeholders. The term "patient focused" does not mean simply being nice to patients or keeping them happy. Patient or customer focus means that the requirements of these groups are the foundation for and drive all work performed by the organization. In turn, organizational processes are designed with the intended result of meeting those patient, customer, and other stakeholder requirements.

Second, "the Voice of the Process defines what you will get from a system" (Wheeler 2000). This phrase defines the concept of *process per-*

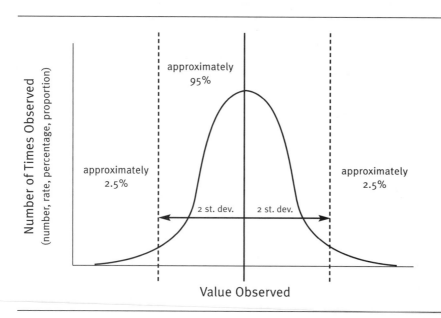

FIGURE 9.2
Frequency
Distribution

formance data. The work of the organization is accomplished through its processes, and the measure of the outcome or process output may be thought of as the "Voice of the Process." Just as the manager listens to the voice of the customer through such avenues as focus groups, satisfaction surveys, regulatory requirements, and reimbursement rates, the manager can listen to the voice of the process through control charts.

"It is management's job to work to bring the Voice of the Process into alignment with the Voice of the Customer. . . . If one is not pleased with the amount of variation shown by the Natural Process Limits, then one must go to work on the system, to change the underlying process rather than setting arbitrary goals, jawboning the workers, or looking for alternative ways of computing the limits" (Wheeler 2000). If process outputs show wide swings over time, the process had been designed in such a manner that it delivers inconsistent rather than steady results. Adding training, working harder, or setting new goals will be ineffective strategies to improve the output of this process.

A manager must be able to recognize the two types of variation illustrated by control charts. *Random variation,* also referred to as noise, is the natural variation present in the process, while *assignable variation,* also referred to as a signal, indicates that a change in the process has occurred. The manager can distinguish random variation as those points that lie within the boundaries of the upper and lower control limits. Assignable variation is present when any of the following situations are seen by the manager (Wheeler 2000):

- when a value is above the upper control limit or below the lower control limit,

FIGURE 9.3
Statistical
Process
Control Chart

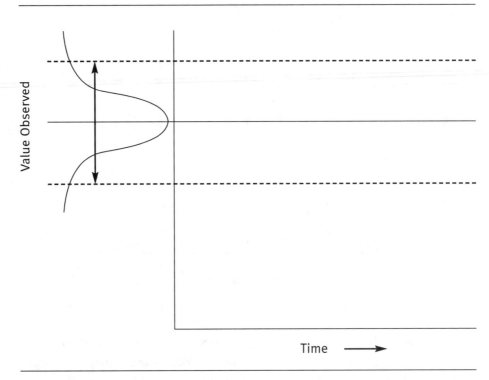

• when three to four successive values lie closer to the control limits than they do to the mean, or
• when eight or more consecutive points lie on the same side of the mean.

The reason that a manager must be able to distinguish between random and assignable variation is that he or she will need to respond differently, depending on the type of variation present. A manager cannot do anything to change the amount of random variation exhibited by the process except to change, redesign, or improve the underlying process itself. Assignable variation results from a distinct cause that may be investigated and identified by the manager. Once identified, the manager may eliminate or simply explain the cause.

Example

The following example illustrates how a manager may integrate statistical process control charts into hospital operations. In this example, the process being studied involves scheduling patient surgeries and allocating staff as needed. The "voice of the customer" includes hospital administration requiring cost-effective use of staffing dollars, physicians requiring the availability of a skilled operating room team, and employees requiring a satisfactory distribution of work hours. Figure 9.4 tracks the number of employee overtime hours for an operating room over four years.

In control charts, it is not uncommon to group data into time periods and to calculate the mean and control limits on the basis of the time periods selected. In this example, the end of the annual budget cycle was a natural cutoff point. As Figure 9.4 shows, each point indicates the actual number of overtime hours worked (y-axis) during each of the 26 pay periods in the calendar year (x-axis). The mean number of overtime hours for the year is shown as the center line, with the upper and lower control limits set at two standard deviations above and below the mean, respectively. In Year 1, Point A and Point B alert the manager to assignable variation. Upon investigation, the manager discovered that, during these two pay periods, in addition to staff absences because of vacation leaves, several staff had also attended professional conferences. Although the scheduling policy limited the number of staff who could be absent for vacation at one time and the number of staff who could be sent to workshops at one time, the policy failed to take into account the two instances of absences. By understanding this root cause, the manager redesigned the scheduling policy to limit the number of staff who could simultaneously be scheduled to be absent for any reason.

The portion of the control chart showing data for Year 2 provides the manager a warning by showing increased variability in how the process is performing, which is indicated by the wider distance between the upper and lower control limits as well as by an increase in the average number of overtime hours per pay period. This pattern in the random variation indicates that the process is not performing as effectively as it was during the previous year. (Note that if the original mean and control limits were extended from Year 1 into Year 2, the consecutive values above the mean alert the manager that something has changed in the process. In this case, patient volumes were increasing, while the scheduling process remained the same.) Point C alerts the manager to assignable variation. When the manager investigated the reason for this variation, she found that it was caused by a large number of employees or their dependents being ill with the flu. Although the manager knew the cause, the variation was expected to be a one-time occurrence, so it was simply explained.

In Year 3, the variability in the process continues to increase to a situation that was just about unmanageable. Growing patient volumes were exacerbated by staff burnout and turnover. At this time, the manager knew that the scheduling process needed to be redesigned, so she requested for a management engineer to analyze the situation and recommend solutions. The interventions (indicated by the arrow) included increasing the baseline number of staff to match the requirements of the growing patient volumes and redistributing staff across shifts to minimize peaks and valleys that had evolved over time to accommodate personnel preferences rather than patient needs.

The performance of the redesigned scheduling process is seen in the Year 4 pay periods. The change resulted in the mean number of overtime

FIGURE 9.4
Control Chart Example

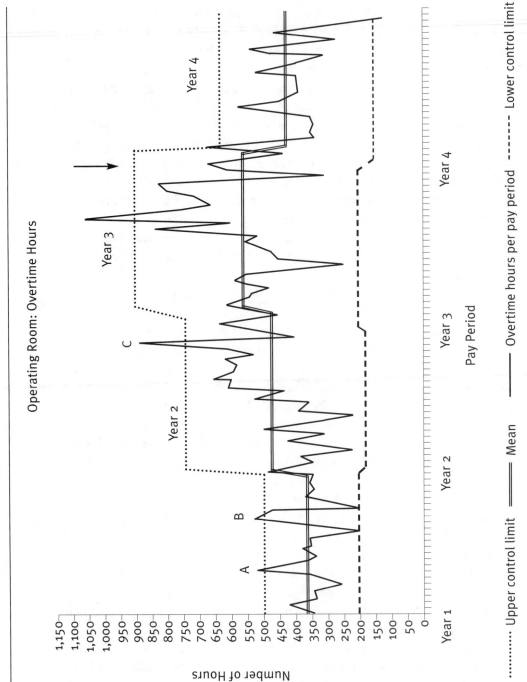

Operating Room: Overtime Hours

hours declining by approximately 30 percent and the variability (standard deviation) declining by about 30 percent. Although not yet as effective as what was seen in Year 1, the new scheduling process was a considerable improvement from the previous two years.

The intentions of this example are to illustrate the difference between random and assignable variation, to describe examples of interventions that a manager may employ, and to illustrate that a control chart can show whether a management change can improve the performance of a process. In this example, the control chart was actually constructed retrospectively to better represent the impact of implementing the management engineer's recommendations. The negative results of the process had enough of an impact on both the manager and the employees to warrant the staffing analysis. Although the manager reviewed overtime hours pay period by pay period, she did not realize the extent to which the process had been out of control until the data were graphed in a control chart. Had the manager been adding the values to the chart as they occurred, the signals could have been observed and action taken in a more timely way.

Conclusion

Performance measurement is essential to performance improvement. Although techniques for collecting, analyzing, and reporting data fall within the quantitative skill set of the organization, translating data into information that managers need to promote performance improvement requires a different and more subtle skill set. This chapter offers measurement examples, insights, and lessons for managers to assist them in better understanding the performance of the systems in which they operate.

The exercise at the end of this chapter provides an opportunity to practice constructing control charts and to understand the "voice of the process." Chapter 10 describes concepts related to initiating and sustaining performance improvement.

Companion Readings

Epstein, R. S., and L. M. Sherwood. 1996. "From Outcomes Research to Disease Management: A Guide for the Perplexed." *Annals of Internal Medicine* 124 (9): 832–37.

Wheeler, D. J. 2000. *Understanding Variation: The Key to Managing Chaos,* 2nd Edition. Knoxville, TN: SPC Press.

References

Aidemark, L. G. 2001. "The Meaning of Balanced Scorecard in the Healthcare Organisation." *Financial Accountability and Management* 17 (1): 23–40.

Baldrige National Quality Program. 2003. *Healthcare Criteria for Performance Excellence.* Gaithersburg, MD: National Institute of Standards and Technology.

Brook, R. H., C. J. Kamberg, and E. McGlynn. 1996. "Health System Reform and Quality." *Journal of the American Medical Association* 276 (6): 476–80.

Chow, C. W., D. Ganulin, O. Teknika, K. Haddad, and J. Williamson. 1998. "The Balanced Scorecard: A Potent Tool for Energizing and Focusing Healthcare Organization Management." *Journal of Healthcare Management* 43 (3): 263–80.

Donabedian, A. 1980. *Explorations in Quality Assessment and Monitoring, Volume I: The Definition of Quality and Approaches to Its Assessment.* Chicago: Health Administration Press.

Fitzgerald, J. F., P. S. Moore, and R. S. Dittus. 1988. "The Care of Elderly Patients with Hip Fracture. Changes Since Implementation of the Prospective Payment System." *New England Journal of Medicine* 319 (21): 1392–97.

Harvard Management Update. 2000. "The Balanced Scorecard's Lessons for Managers." *Harvard Management Update* 5 (10): 4–5.

Inamdar, N., R. S. Kaplan, and M. Bower. 2002. "Applying the Balanced Scorecard in Healthcare Provider Organizations." *Journal of Healthcare Management* 47 (3): 179–95.

Inamdar, N., R. S. Kaplan, M. L. Jones, and R. Menitoff. 2000. "The Balanced Scorecard: A Strategic Management System for Multi-Sector Collaboration and Strategy Implementation." *Quality Management in Healthcare* 8 (4): 21–39.

Jason, O. 2001. "The Balanced Scorecard: An Integrative Approach to Performance Evaluation." *Healthcare Financial Management* 55 (5): 42–46.

Kaplan, R. S., and D. P. Norton. 1996. *The Balanced Scorecard: Translating Strategy into Action.* Boston: Harvard Business School Press.

———. 1993. "Putting the Balanced Scorecard to Work." *Harvard Business Review* 71 (5): 134–39.

———. 1992. "The Balanced Scorecard—Measures that Drive Performance." *Harvard Business Review* 70 (1): 71–79.

Kelly, D. L., S. L. Pestotnik, M. C. Coons, and J. W. Lelis. 1997. "Reengineering a Surgical Service Line: Focusing on Core Process Improvement." *American Journal of Medical Quality.* 12 (2): 120–29.

Nelson, E. C., J. J. Mohr, P. B. Batalden, and S. K. Plume. 1996. "Improving Healthcare, Part 1: The Clinical Value Compass." *Joint Commission Journal on Quality Improvement* 22 (4): 243–58.

Wheeler, D. J. 2000. *Understanding Variation: The Key to Managing Chaos,* 2nd Edition. Knoxville, TN: SPC Press.

Zelman, W. N., D. Blazer, J. M. Glover, P. Bumgarner, and L. Cancilla. 1999. "Issues for Academic Health Centers to Consider Before Implementing a Balanced-Scorecard Effort." *Academic Medicine* 74 (12): 1269–77.

Exercise

Objective:

- To practice presenting data in a statistical process control chart format
- To practice interpreting data presented in a statistical process control chart format

Instructions:

For each of the following data sets:

1. Graph the data in control chart format.
2. Set your control limits by using the mean ±2 standard deviations.
3. Review your control chart.
4. Answer the questions for that data set.

Data Set 1

You are researching a paper on teenage smoking for one of your classes. You come across a newspaper column with the following headline: "Teen Use Turns Upward." The column goes on to say that the percentage of high school seniors who smoked daily was 17.3 percent two years ago and 19.0 percent last year. You happen to have data from another class that show teenage smoking rates for the past ten years. You plot all ten years on a control chart. What does your control chart tell you about the conclusion stated in the newspaper headline?

Ten years of teen smoking rates are shown below. Those years referred to in the newspaper are marked with an asterisk (*). The mean and standard deviation for the ten years are also provided.

Year 1	18.8	Mean	18.5
Year 2	19.6	St. dev.	0.80
Year 3	18.7		
Year 4	18.6		
Year 5	17.1		
Year 6	18.9		
Year 7	19.2		
Year 8	18.2		
*Year 9	17.3		
*Year 10	19.0		

Data Set 2

You have been in your new job as a manager at a pharmaceutical company for one month. You have been assigned to the unit that is making vaccines for next year's flu season, and you have been given the last four weeks' production volume statistics: 23.2, 23.5, 23.1, and 27.7. Your boss is concerned about having the production capacity to meet the increased predictions for the upcoming flu season. On the basis of his analysis, weekly production volumes will have to average 27.5 to meet demand. What do you tell him about what the process is able to deliver? What recommendations do you make?

Twenty-two weeks of production volumes are shown below. The mean and standard deviation are also provided

Week	Production Volume	Mean	24.4
		St. dev.	2.3
1	21.6		
2	23.9		
3	23.3		
4	22.6		
5	28.8		
6	22.7		
7	23.8		
8	22.8		
9	28.7		
10	22.9		
11	24.2		
12	23.2		
13	28.6		
14	22.8		
15	23.9		
16	23.2		
17	23.7		
18	28.5		
19	23.2		
20	23.5		
21	23.1		
22	27.7		

Data Set 3

You are attending a quality improvement workshop and are browsing around the poster session. Your eye catches a presentation about congestive heart failure, and you see the average length of stay data displayed in control chart format, which contains the data presented below. Describe any signals or noise that you observe in the control chart. List three to five questions that you would ask the presenters so that you may better understand the signals.

The average length of hospital stay in days is shown below. Determine the time interval for calculating the mean and standard deviation for your control chart before performing the calculations and plotting the data.

Month	Days
Year 1	
Jan	6.1
Feb	6.5
Mar	6.8
Apr	5.9
May	6.3
June	6.4
July	6.6
Aug	6.3
Sept	6.2
Oct	6.4
Nov	6.5
Dec	6.8
Year 2	
Jan	6.2
Feb	5.4
Mar	5.6
Apr	5.5
May	5.2
June	5
July	4.8
Aug	4.6
Sept	4.4
Oct	4.2
Nov	4.5
Dec	4

ORGANIZATIONAL TRACTION

Objectives

- To describe the elements of organizational traction
- To describe the importance of organizational traction in initiating and sustaining ongoing performance improvement
- To gain an appreciation for the need to define current reality

When an unexpected snow catches a warm-weather city by surprise, cars may be seen slipping and sliding on the roads. A bicyclist uses one type of bike for riding on the street and a different type for riding on mountain trails. A ski racer carefully chooses his or her wax to avoid being slowed down by the snow. A car hydroplanes on the highway during an intense rainstorm.

Each of these situations is influenced by traction. The ability to understand and manage traction is the difference between safely getting to work on time and sliding off the road, getting stuck in the mud and having a great ride, winning a ski race and losing it, and arriving safely at a destination or reeling out of control.

Traction is that force that allows something to stay connected to a surface. It may be intentionally increased to attach to the surface (e.g., with specially designed tires) or intentionally decreased to detach from the surface (e.g., with types of ski wax). The force of traction is also exerted when something is being drawn; pulleys, cranes, and winches enable a person to draw, lift, or move something that he or she would be unable to otherwise. The same can be said of organizations. An understanding of organizational traction and organizational "pulleys" allows managers to initiate and sustain movement in quality, change, and performance improvement efforts and to stay the course toward the goal.

A common question that managers and students alike ask when discussing improvement efforts is, "How do you get people to change?" In his classic *Harvard Business Review* article, Frederick Herzberg (2003) introduces the phrase "KITA"—an acronym for "kick in the 'pants'." He offered KITA as one approach to motivating employees and job enrichment (i.e., designing meaningful work that employees desire to do) as another. Likewise with initiating or motivating organizational change: the manager may choose a push strategy, or the manager may choose strategies that manage traction in the work environment to draw employees along a path of change and improvement.

This chapter explores two types of organizational traction. The first type helps managers to initiate change—that is, getting a car going on a slippery surface rather than having it sitting there spinning its wheels. The second type helps managers to maintain an ongoing environment of quality and performance improvement—that is, once the car gets going, keeping it moving.

Initiating Change

The Animal Control Services team at a county health department recognized that the community had a huge problem. In the past several years, there had been an increase in county pet populations, stray animals, and animal bites as well as the reemergence of rabies after years of being free of it. The team made some progress when it instituted a 100 percent sterilization requirement for adopted animals. Although they offered pet sterilization to any animal currently being adopted, the process was cumbersome. As a result, many owners did not follow-up once they took their new pet home or decided against adopting altogether. The team had an idea to redesign the pet adoption process that would enable the pets to be sterilized before they left the animal shelter rather than have the new owner assume the responsibility.

The challenge was that their new plan would require some allocation of funds from the county commissioners. The team realized that this was an important public health issue; however, they were faced with the problem of how to communicate their sense of urgency to an audience with little knowledge of the issue. Faced with only five minutes on the county commissioner's agenda, the team decided on the following approach: present the facts and share the vision of a successful program. The veterinarian director of the team started the presentation with the following:

> Start with one female dog . . . in the first year, she produces an average of eight puppies, four of them females . . . in the second year, production of first and second generation females is 40 pups, 20 of them females . . . in the third year, production from three generations of females is 200 pups . . . in the fourth year, production from four generations is 1000 . . . and so on . . . by the eighth generation, this one female pup has resulted in the production of 625,000 puppies!!!" (McNeil et al. 2002)

After the veterinarian gave a few statistics on animal bites and rabies and a brief overview of the plan for the new pet adoption process, the county commissioners were sold. A local reporter concluded a column describing the Animal Control Services's proposal with the comment, "The only question at this point would seem to be, is it possible to move faster . . . ?" (*Wilmington Morning Star* 2002)

Animal Control Services understood how to use traction to engage stakeholders, gain support for their vision, and jump-start their improvement effort. First, they stated the facts, which in this case were the reproductive capacity of one female puppy and the health consequences of pet overpopulation. Next, they offered their vision of a process. Finally, by clearly revealing the performance gap between what currently existed and what was possible, the team used the concept of creative tension to establish the traction needed to get their effort moving forward (McNeil et al. 2002).

Creative Tension

Just as the medical specialty of surgery consists of subspecialties like neurosurgery, orthopedic surgery, and plastic surgery, the field of systems thinking also consists of subfields. One of these subfields is called *structural dynamics*. Tension resolution is the fundamental building block in structural dynamics (Fritz 1996). When a difference exists between one thing and another, the resulting discrepancy creates the tendency toward movement. One type of tension found in organizations is called *creative tension,* which is formed by the discrepancy between an organization's current level of performance and its desired level and vision for the future.

The rubber band metaphor has been used to illustrate the concept of creative tension (Senge 1990). Think of holding a rubber band, with one end in each hand and one hand above the other. Stretch the rubber band, and feel the tension of the pull. Think of the higher hand as vision—that is, the desired future state of the organization. Think of the lower hand as current reality—that is, the current level of the organization's performance. The tension may be released from the rubber band by only two ways.

The first way to relieve tension is to let go of the end clasped by the lower hand. As the tension is released, the rubber band is drawn to the top hand. The greater the tension, the faster and more strongly the rubber band will snap. In organizations, this tension resolution may be seen as being drawn toward a vision. The second way to relieve tension is to let go of the end clasped by the higher hand. As the tension is released, the rubber band is drawn to the bottom hand. In organizations, this tension resolution may be seen as simply maintaining the status quo or stagnating performance, despite well-intentioned efforts to improve.

When organizational change and performance are viewed through a systems perspective, tension resolution is the key traction tool for changing behavior. The essential elements for creative tension to be present in an organization are current reality, vision, and an actual or perceived gap between the two. Managers may consciously create or make visible discrepancies in the organization to leverage the resulting tendency toward movement.

Current Reality

Establishing creative tension requires some sort of common, objective description of current reality. The description may range from a very simple evaluation to an in-depth organizational assessment. Without some objective depiction of the current situation of the organization, individuals may be left to create their own pictures of current reality based on their own limited information sets. Without a shared understanding of current reality, the manager's ability to take advantage of creative tension is limited.

Organizational assessment and diagnosis may be more familiar to strategic planners who have used SWOT analysis (*S*trengths, *W*eaknesses, *O*pportunities, *T*hreats) or to organizational development professionals than to managers. However, the concept and practice of assessment offers a valuable way for managers to document, communicate, and promote a shared understanding of current reality. An *organizational assessment* or *self-assessment* simply refers to a systematic or repeatable method of examining the organization for its strengths and performance gaps. An organizational self-assessment conducted at regular intervals (e.g., annually, biannually) provides managers with the opportunity and impetus to systematically reexamine, document, and communicate current reality relative to desired organizational activities, strategies, and performance results. In Chapter 5, several systems models were introduced, including the Baldrige National Quality Award Healthcare Criteria for Performance Excellence. The Baldrige model may be best known for its national award, but it is also an important guide for organizational self-assessment.

As managers begin to understand creative tension, they will also begin to see that a performance measurement system is a vital management tool to describe, monitor, and communicate current reality. In the absence of performance measures, those within the organization will define currently reality on the basis of their own mental models, knowledge, and previous experiences. As a result, some may hold an inflated view of the organization's current reality, while others may hold a disproportionately negative view. The net effect is the absence of a shared understanding of current reality, which leads to a shared understanding of the performance gap that is necessary for creative tension. Without creative tension, no need exists for tension resolution and, in turn, no traction for change.

Vision

Vision plays a role in leadership (Kotter 2001; Kouzes and Posner 1987; Tichey 1997), personal effectiveness (Covey 1990), organizational effectiveness (Senge 1990), art (Fritz 1989), and even survival (Frankl 1962). Vision is also an essential element in creative tension and in creating traction for change.

Visions may be found at a variety of levels within healthcare. The Office of Disease Prevention and Health Promotion, through the U.S.

Department of Health and Human Services's Healthy People Initiatives, offers an overall vision for the nation's health:

> . . . regardless of age, gender, race or ethnicity, income, education, geographic location, disability, and sexual orientation—every person in every community across the Nation deserves equal access to comprehensive, culturally competent, community-based healthcare systems that are committed to serving the needs of the individual and promoting community health. (Healthy People 2010 2003a)

This vision provides a common direction for diverse groups that share the interest of improving health and healthcare within the United States. The vision is further described by defining specific areas of focus, such as access, environmental health, public health infrastructure, and infectious diseases, and by defining ideal performance in a variety of health indicators. The ten health indicators—physical activity, overweight and obesity, tobacco use, substance abuse, responsible sexual behavior, mental health, injury and violence, environmental quality, immunization, and access to healthcare—provide direction for groups to individualize their own community visions within the larger national context (Healthy People 2010 2003b).

Organizations often have an overall vision for the future. Managers may also use the concept of vision in a variety of ways and at various levels within the organization. Managers may have visions for their careers, for their own professional contribution to quality healthcare, or for their ideal departments or service areas. Managers may ask a team to describe its ideal vision for a particular work process or process of care. When managers understand that vision is an essential element of creative tension, they will also realize that vision is essential to quality management and organizational effectiveness.

In creating a vision, describing characteristics of the ideal future state is helpful. Questions that physicians may pose when creating a vision for their own office practice may include the following:

If my practice was recognized as one of the best in the country . . .
- What would patients and families say about the care they received?
- What would patients and families say about their interactions with me? With my office staff?
- What would my colleagues around the country say about my practice?
- What processes in my office would colleagues most want to emulate?
- How do I and my office staff feel after a day's work?
- If a prominent journal or newspaper were writing about my office practice, what would the article say?

When creating a vision, one should not be limited by what is possible or what is not possible. By defining characteristics of the ideal future rather than ideal interventions, a manager may balance describing an ideal future with present constraints. Healthcare workers often respond with

"We would have that new computer system" or "We would totally remodel the office" when asked about their ideal unit or office. However, financial constraints may not allow for these expenditures at the time, which makes constructing the vision an exercise in futility rather than a chance to describe a future ideal state. Rather than "We would have that new computer system," the ideal answer can be, "We have streamlined, user-friendly documentation and communication mechanisms in place for both our internal office operations and for our patients." Rather than "We would totally remodel the office," the ideal answer can be, "Patients will find a clean, accessible, comfortable, and relaxing office environment that respects their privacy and confidentiality."

By defining characteristics of the ideal future rather than ideal interventions that are more specific to the way things are now, opportunities for creative and flexible ways of achieving the vision while working within the constraints of the situation may be enhanced.

Maintaining an Ongoing Environment of Quality and Performance Improvement

In Chapter 6, the concept of mental models was introduced as a deeply ingrained way of thinking that influences how a person sees and understands the world and that influences how a person acts. *Context* is a concept closely related to mental models and is defined as "the unquestioning assumptions through which all experience is filtered" (Davis 1982). In this book, the term *mental models* refer to an individual's assumptions, while the term *context* refers to organizational assumptions that guide how the organization defines itself and how it operates.

Context

Let us now explore two illustrations of context to better understand the subtle difference between mental models and context. Here is the first illustration:

> Consider this analogy. You inherit your grandmother's house. Unknown to you is one peculiarity: all the light fixtures have bulbs that give off a blue rather than yellow light. You find that you don't like the feel of the rooms and spend a lot of time and money repainting walls, reupholstering furniture, and replacing carpets. You never seem to get it quite right, but nonetheless, you rationalize that at least it is improving with each thing you do. Then one day you notice the blue light bulbs and change them. Suddenly, all that you fixed is broken.
>
> Context is like the color of the light, not the objects in the room. Context colors everything in the corporation. More accurately, the context alters what we see, usually without our being aware of it. (Goss, Pascale, and Athos 1993)

An external community focus may represent one operating context for a healthcare organization, while an internal organizational focus may represent a different operating context. Management decisions about resource allocation, prevention, or continuum-of-care issues will differ depending on the context or assumptions about the organization's focus or role in the community.

Consider this second illustration of context, which suggests a corollary to the concept: content.

> Most parents have dreams for their children. Some want their children to be doctors, some musicians, and all want them to be healthy, wealthy, and wise. These are parents raising their children by focusing on content. Following in a father's footsteps, or in the footsteps father never had and therefore wants for his son, are well-known examples of this approach. Other parents, however, raise their children by focusing on context. In Helen Keller's famous phrase, their dream is, "be all you can be." The orientation here is to "parent" the context and let the child discover the content. (Davis 1982)

As stated in the illustration, managers may also find themselves facing the dichotomy of which—context or content—to manage. One may think of the distinctions between context and content as they are demonstrated in Figure 10.1. The boundary of the circle is the context; the inside of the circle is the content (Davis 1982).

Historically, healthcare managers have been promoted on the basis of their content expertise: an excellent pharmacist becomes the manager of the entire pharmacy department; an excellent engineer becomes the manager of the facilities maintenance department; or an excellent clinician becomes a department, division, or unit manager. These managerial roles generally include directly supervising both the people and the work.

Today, the organizations, environments, processes, and technologies in healthcare are so complex that managers cannot be experts on managing and on the content of the work that needs to be managed. Managers' roles will increasingly move away from managing content to managing context. This means that employees with fundamental knowledge of the work itself will carry out and improve their work processes, while managers will ensure that employees have the appropriate tools, information, knowledge, and competency to effectively do their jobs and deliver quality services and products.

Managing context also suggests managing the boundaries of the system, which may be a unit, a department, an office practice, a service line, or an entire organization. Boundaries may be defined in terms of scope of work, decision-making authority, or accountability. The manager may set or reset the boundaries on the basis of environmental conditions and other organizational considerations. In a department with a high ratio of experienced

FIGURE 10.1
Context

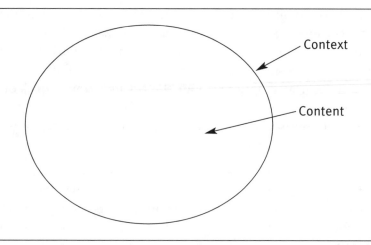

employees, the manager may expand the boundary so that staff are more autonomous in their decision making. However, in a department composed of a young or inexperienced staff, the manager may tighten the boundaries of decision making until staff gains knowledge, ability, and confidence in their own decision-making skills.

Managing the boundaries of the system also suggests that the managers not only define their own areas of responsibility but also the interfaces that occur at the boundaries. As organizations shifted to a structure of self-directed work teams, the supervisory role also shifted to one of "boundary manager" (Orsburn et al. 1990). This meant that, rather than supervising individuals, the supervisor helped teams to interact with each other as needed to coordinate work, communicate information, or resolve problems. Likewise, effectively managing context requires an awareness and understanding of the interfaces with other systems both within and outside of the organization. In the example described in Chapter 4 (trade-offs), the manager who anticipated unintended consequences of reducing hospital length of stay and proactively worked with the nursing homes demonstrates an awareness and understanding of the interface of acute care and nursing home care.

The best way to become aware of context and to then draw the appropriate boundary for the system is by asking the right questions (Davis 1982). For managers, the key to asking the right questions is to not be afraid to challenge current assumptions; otherwise, the answers to the questions will simply be a restatement of what is already known rather than truly seeking to understand and explore what is beyond the current boundary of knowledge or awareness. Unless managers and other healthcare professionals challenge context, the creation of innovative improvements and excellent performance in healthcare systems will be limited. For this reason, the common theme of Section III is to offer the manager structured ways to test underlying assumptions and ask new questions about goals, purpose, measurement, implementation, and teams.

Context and Vision

A common cliché in healthcare is "change is a given," and the same can be said of ambiguity. Already present to some degree, ambiguity and uncertainty will continue to increase as inherent characteristics of the environments in which healthcare organizations operate. Integrating vision and context can help managers create a work environment to more effectively deal with ambiguity.

A young child putting together a puzzle illustrates how vision and context are related. The child empties the puzzle pieces from the box and then props up the box to see a picture of what the puzzle is supposed to look like when it is completed. He then sorts the pieces: one group contains pieces with a straight edge or a corner shape, and one group contains the odd shapes. When asked why, the child replies, "To make the outside first." Once the outer edge of the puzzle is assembled, he goes about fitting the rest of the pieces, knowing that each piece will eventually have its own place in the picture.

The manager's role in establishing vision may be thought of as making sure everyone in the organization has the ability to see the entire picture—that is, what the puzzle would look like when it is completed. The manager's role in setting the boundaries or context of the system may be thought of as putting together the outer edge of the puzzle. The images or shapes of the individual pieces may be thought of as the content, which is what goes on or what is done within the organization. Although there is much ambiguity at first about where the individual pieces should go, enough information is available to continue the task of building the puzzle or, in the manager's case, moving toward the vision of the future.

Conclusion

The key to sustainable change in organizations is to identify and address underlying structures, as described in Chapter 6. The key to initiating movement toward improvement is to address tension resolution. The key to maintaining an environment of ongoing performance improvement is to address context. These three activities fall within the manager's domain of responsibility; addressing the content—the actual care, work, and technical process—falls within the domain of responsibility of the frontline workers and care providers.

In clinical services, the physical exam or annual checkup is a commonplace activity. The exercise at the end of this chapter continues to explore the value of an organizational assessment in defining current reality by comparing it to a physical exam. Once the concept of traction is understood, the focus of implementing changes and improvements shifts from overcoming staff resistance to supporting staff success. Chapter 11 describes several implementation lessons that may enhance a manager's ability to support staff and, in turn, successfully integrate improvements into operations of the organization.

Companion Readings

Heifetz, R. A., and D. L. Laurie. 2001. "The Work of Leadership." *Harvard Business Review* 79 (11): 131–40.

Davis, S. M. 1982. "Transforming Organizations: The Key to Strategy Is Context." *Organizational Dynamics* 10 (3): 64–80.

Fritz, R. 1989. *The Path of Least Resistance: Learning to Become the Creative Force in Your Own Life*, Chapter 9. New York: Ballantine.

References

Covey, S. R. 1990. *The Seven Habits of Highly Effective People*. New York: Simon and Schuster.

Davis, S. M. 1982. "Transforming Organizations: The Key to Strategy is Context." *Organizational Dynamics* 10 (3): 64–80.

Frankl, V. E. 1962. *Man's Search for Meaning: An Introduction to Logotherapy*. Boston: Beacon Press.

Fritz, R. 1996. *Corporate Tides: The Inescapable Laws of Organizational Structure*. San Francisco: Berrett-Koehler Publishers.

———. 1989. *The Path of Least Resistance: Learning to Become the Creative Force in Your Own Life*. New York: Ballantine.

Goss, T., R. Pascale, and A. Athos. 1993. "The Reinvention Roller Coaster: Risking the Present for a Powerful Future." *Harvard Business Review* 71 (6): 97–108.

Healthy People 2010. 2003a. "A Systematic Approach to Health Improvement: Objectives." [Online information; retrieved 2/20/03]. http://www.health.gov/healthypeople/Document/html/uih/uih_2.htm #obj.

———. 2003b. "Healthy People 2010 Home Page." [Online information; retrieved February 20, 2003]. http://www.health.gov/healthypeople.

Herzberg, F. 2003. "One More Time: How Do You Motivate Employees?" *Harvard Business Review* 81 (1): 87–96.

Kotter, J. P. 2001. "What Leaders Really Do." *Harvard Business Review* 79 (11): 85–90.

Kouzes, J. M., and B. Z. Posner. 1987. *The Leadership Challenge: How to Keep Getting Extraordinary Things Done in Organizations*. San Francisco: Jossey-Bass.

McNeil, J. P., D. Brown, D. Howard, B. McClure, and G. R. Weedon. 2002. "Sterilization Protects Animals and You." Presentation to the University of North Carolina at Chapel Hill Management Academy for Public Health, April 25.

Orsburn, J. D., L. Moran, E. Musselwhite, and J. H. Zenger. 1990. *Self-Directed Work Teams: The New American Challenge*. Homewood, IL: Business One Irwin.

Senge, P. M. 1990. *The Fifth Discipline: The Art and Practice of the Learning Organization*. New York: Doubleday Currency.

Tichey, N. M. 1997. *The Leadership Engine: How Winning Companies Build Leaders at Every Level*. New York: Harper Collins Publishers, Inc.

Wilmington Morning Star. 2002. "Saving Pets and Taxpayers." (January 7): page 6A.

Exercise

Objective: To gain an appreciation for a regular assessment of current reality in an organization

Instructions:

1. An integral activity in any healthcare provider-patient encounter involves the physical examination, checkup, or assessment. This exercise will examine what may be learned about the organizational examination, checkup, or assessment from this routine clinical practice.

    For questions 1a through 1e, you may choose to record your responses on the Assessment Worksheet below or one similar to it.

    a. Describe the purpose of an annual physical examination. You may answer from a provider or patient point of view. You may discuss a physical examination, a well-child checkup, or even a dental appointment.

    b. Describe the general sequence of events that occur during this examination.

    c. How do you (if you answered as a provider) or the provider (if you answered as a patient) know what to do to complete the examination?

    d. Describe why the examination is done in this particular way.

    e. Answer the same questions for an organization, and fill in the "Organizational Checkup" column in the worksheet below.

    f. On the basis of your responses to the above questions, describe why managers should or should not perform organizational checkups on a routine basis.

Assessment Worksheet

	Physical Checkup	Organizational Checkup
Purpose		
Sequence of events		
How do you know what to do?		
Why is it done this way?		

CHAPTER

11

IMPLEMENTATION LESSONS

Objectives

- To address operational considerations related to implementing improvements
- To introduce an implementation framework for managers
- To gain an appreciation for the influence of mental models on implementation

Consider two approaches to purchasing a new home. Every day for a week, Person A searched the real-estate advertisements in the newspapers. His diligent search yielded some properties that he was interested in, so he called a realtor for a tour of each. After seeing a certain property, he immediately knew that this was his "perfect house." The realtor referred him to a mortgage company to work out the financing. Person A was confident that no problem would arise because, based on his own calculations, his salary could cover the monthly payments. But then he received the bad news: he could not qualify for the financing. Payments on a new car bought six months earlier, outstanding credit card bills from a recent vacation, and a small savings account all worked against him. Person A only qualified for a loan that was much smaller than he anticipated and needed for his dream home.

Person A's coworker, Person B, has a hobby of scanning the real-estate news. For years, Person B has been watching trends, and through that he has identified a particular area of the city in which he would like to purchase a house. Based on the average housing prices in that area, Person B calculated what he would need for a down payment as well as for monthly mortgage payments. He systematically accumulated the funds for the down payment, made sure he paid his credit cards' balances down to zero every month, and prequalified with a mortgage company. Although most of his friends and coworkers drove brand new cars, his car was five years old but completely paid. When Person B's "perfect house" came on the market, he was the first to see it and was able to complete the purchase without a problem. When Person A overheard Person B talking about his new address, Person A could not believe it; he wondered, "How could he possibly afford that place when he makes the same salary as I do?"

The answer to Person A's question is that these coworkers used two entirely different approaches to planning and implementing their processes

167

for house buying. Person A used an approach called *forward planning,* which involves taking one step at a time and not knowing the next step until after the previous step is completed. Person B used an approach called *reverse planning* (Dorner 1996), which involves defining the desired end result—in this case, his ideal house—and then working backward to determine a practical or logical starting point to the step-by-step process of getting to the end result. In reverse planning, each step is a necessary precondition to the next step. By planning in this manner, Person B could make purposeful choices (e.g., not buying a new car, reducing his credit card debt) that would help him toward, rather than become barriers to, the end goal of purchasing his ideal house.

Similar approaches have been described in the literature. Habit number two in *The Seven Habits of Highly Effective People* by Stephen Covey (1990) advises to "begin with the end in mind." The "solution after next principle" from *Breakthrough Thinking: The Seven Principles of Creative Problem Solving* indicates that more effective solutions may be generated "by working backward from an ideal target solution for the future" (Nadler and Hibino 1994).

This chapter introduces an implementation framework derived from the common themes of these three approaches. First, however, operational considerations for implementing improvement efforts are described and the relationship between mental models and successful implementation are explored.

Operational Considerations

In addition to the particulars of the intended intervention, managers should take into account the measurement system, unintended consequences, and staff issues when planning for the implementation of an improvement or change effort.

Measurement System

"How will you know if the change is an improvement?" (Langley et al. 1996) is a fundamental question managers should ask about any improvement effort. Chapter 7 illustrated an example of how a surgical services manager first set general goals to be able to establish overall direction and specific goals. The manager's first goal was to design and implement the performance measurement system. This goal took a while to achieve because data had to be collected from a variety of sources and from different electronic databases, but it taught the manager the importance of having a measurement system in place as the foundation for understanding the impact of future interventions, whether for a specific process improvement (e.g., preoperative laboratory tests) or for an intervention affecting the entire department (e.g., redesigned governance structure) (Kelly et al. 1997).

Managers must be able to distinguish between measuring the impact of a single intervention and measuring the overall performance of the system (e.g., department, service, organization) over which the manager is responsible. Unlike a clinical trial, where the researchers are closely manipulating the variables to be tested, the numerous interrelated variables at work in complex healthcare organizations make it difficult for managers to determine the precise impact of a single intervention. The characteristics of dynamic complexity (see Chapter 4) and the subsequent need to use multiple goals when operating in complex systems (see Chapter 7) suggest that measures of a single change are only one component of an overall performance measurement system.

A performance measurement system should be the very first step of implementation, not only because of its role in describing, monitoring, and communicating current reality and progress toward the vision (see Chapter 10) but also because it provides information about the influence of improvement interventions on the behavior of the overall system. If a measurement system is already in place, then the manager/team/organization may continue with implementing operational and other improvements. Although not typically thought of as an implementation intervention, a performance measurement system may be viewed by managers as a management improvement intervention.

If the manager does not already have an effective performance measurement system in place, planning other improvements may continue; however, implementation should be delayed until the measurement system is designed and put into place. If customer and stakeholder requirements are drivers of improvement, the general direction of performance requirements should be known, and general rather than specific goals may initially be set. In other words, the manager desires some measure to improve, and improvement may be described in terms of going down (e.g., costs or cycle times) or going up (e.g., patient satisfaction). Once a means to measure the impact of the intervention is in place, managers or teams may implement the intervention and monitor the performance in relation to the goal. As ongoing data are collected and thus provide more information about performance, more specific goals may be set.

This approach to measurement may sound counterintuitive to those accustomed to measurement within the context of clinical research or other approaches that require accumulating baseline data trends over time. Derived from a management and performance improvement mental model on measurement, the performance measurement approach described in the preceding paragraph takes into account the complex nature of healthcare organizations and offers managers a way to reduce the improvement-process cycle time, which is the time from when the improvement is initiated to the time that results are seen. Note that management data must demonstrate reliability and validity; however, because the intended use is to monitor and improve performance, other data characteristics (e.g., sample size, bias definition, data-collection methods, the relationship of the data to the hypothesis) may differ from data used for other purposes (James 2001).

Unintended Consequences

In a large tertiary hospital, one improvement effort was aimed at decreasing the amount of time patients spent on the ventilator after coronary bypass surgery. A patient's progress toward recovery could be greatly enhanced if less time was spent connected to the ventilator. The improvement team thoughtfully took into account the upstream influences on the patient recovery process by inviting operating room staff and an anesthesiologist to be members of the improvement team.

After bypass surgery, when a patient met the required clinical criteria, he or she was transferred from the intensive care unit (ICU), where each nurse cared for one to two patients, to the acute care patient care unit, where each nurse cared for four to six patients. After the new ICU protocol was put into place, patients who had coronary bypass surgery began arriving in the acute care unit a day earlier than usual. Although these patients were not on ventilators anymore, the extra day of recovery made a difference in other aspects of their care. As a result, the patients arrived sicker and required a special nurse ratio of one nurse to two to three patients, rather than the typical one nurse to four to six patients. The acute care unit was finding itself short staffed on numerous occasions. Although the same number of nurses was being scheduled, the higher patient acuity led to the unit's understaffing.

After several weeks, the acute care unit nurses realized that a change had been made in the ICU's postoperative process. It took the nurse manager several months to hire the required staff to meet the new acuity demands, during which time the existing nurses remained short staffed and overworked.

Chapter 9 introduced the concept of unintended consequences, which are important considerations for managers and teams when implementing improvement efforts within their own work areas, departments, and organizations. Anticipating, identifying, measuring, and proactively managing unintended consequences should be considered in any implementation plan. Figure 11.1 illustrates how this ICU improvement team may have identified unintended consequences by asking not only "Who affects our process" but also "Who is affected by our process?"

Staff Issues

The manager's responsibility is to ensure that the appropriate organizational conditions are in place to enhance successful implementation. Managers may do this by asking themselves the question, "What needs to happen to ensure success?" The following considerations serve as starting points.

First, depending on the scope of the improvement effort, the manager may need to provide a staffing "cushion," which means that he or she

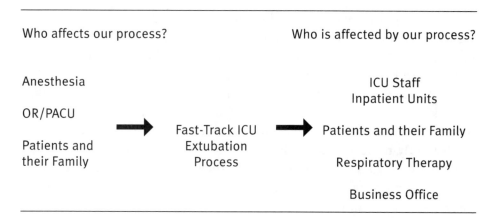

FIGURE 11.1
Anticipating
Unintended
Consequences

Who affects our process?		Who is affected by our process?
Anesthesia		ICU Staff
		Inpatient Units
OR/PACU	Fast-Track ICU	
	Extubation	Patients and their Family
Patients and	Process	
their Family		Respiratory Therapy
		Business Office

has to overstaff initially. Adapting to something new and learning new processes or roles takes time and planning ahead; the manager must not only acknowledge but also actively support the staff's learning curves. Second, the manager may need to negotiate for the necessary short-term budget or productivity variances required for the transition period; however, the long-term benefits to productivity should compensate for the short-term variance.

Third, managers must also ask, "Do staff members have the knowledge and skills required to succeed?" The manager, again, is responsible for ensuring that all staff have the necessary information, training, and tools to enable them to successfully implement improvements. No matter how elegant the solution, inadequately prepared staff can undermine the success of implementation.

Relationship Between Mental Models and Implementation

Although a cliché, the phrase "actions speak louder than words" represents an important consideration when implementing improvement efforts. The idea is also captured in the phrase, "Process and content are inseparable" (Kofman and Senge 1993). This concept means that how a manager goes about improving is equally as important as what the manager chooses to improve.

The term *content* refers to an actual intervention, technique, or process improvement. The term *process* refers to all of the steps involved in

- identifying, studying, and evaluating a problem;
- initiating, organizing, selecting, and facilitating the solution-generating process;
- communicating and preparing staff to implement the intervention; and
- measuring, evaluating, refining, and sustaining performance.

Setting effective goals and clarifying purpose guide managers and teams in content decisions to improve performance results, but an awareness of the influence of mental models may guide the manager in process decisions to improve implementation results.

As described in Chapter 6, mental models shape an individual's actions, and, likewise, an individual's actions provide clues to the underlying mental models. For example, a manager that promotes empowerment verbally but holds tightly to decisions and information sends the message through his actions that he does not promote empowerment. Management interventions and change processes may also be considered activities that provide clues to underlying mental models and that, in turn, send messages to staff. An improvement team may be told to "share opinions openly" or that "all opinions are welcome." However, if team members are rebuked each time a contrasting idea is offered, the team quickly realizes that the process is operating from a mental model that in fact does not welcome all opinions.

Framework for Implementation

Figure 11.2 illustrates a conceptual framework for implementation, referred to in this book as *breakthrough vision, incremental implementation* (Kelly et al. 1997).

Similar diagrams resembling a flight of stairs have been used to illustrate the incremental nature of continuous improvement of existing technology as compared with breakthrough technologies. Figure 11.3 shows an example of how the writing process has improved over time, beginning with paper-and-pen approaches on the left, followed by incremental improvements to paper-and-pen methods. The first large step represents the invention of the typewriter (A), which is then followed by additional improvements to the typewriter (B). The second large step represents the breakthrough technology of computerized word processing (C).

A challenge for healthcare managers is that breakthrough technologies are most often associated with clinical breakthroughs in diagnosis (e.g., magnetic resonance imaging), intervention (e.g., laparoscopic surgery techniques), treatment (e.g., new drugs), or prevention (e.g., polio vaccination). Although specific technology breakthroughs are available that may enhance performance in the management domain (e.g., electronic information systems), management breakthroughs that influence organizational performance are most often associated with the environment in which the clinical technologies may be used. Management breakthroughs may be seen (1) in areas such as philosophy, approaches, and tools that enable managers to promote innovations in the operating environment and (2) in work processes that enable patients to fully realize the benefit of advancements in clinical technology.

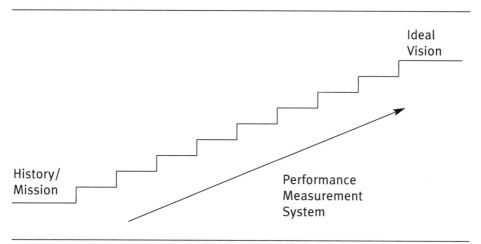

FIGURE 11.2
Breakthrough
Vision,
Incremental
Implementation

Figure 11.4 illustrates the assumptions on which the breakthrough vision, incremental implementation framework is based. Rather than the breakthrough resulting from a technical invention, the breakthrough is defined through the vision and/or context of the department, service, or organization (A). Refinements or adjustments may be made according to changes in the environment or customer/stakeholder expectations (B). The vision and/or context may require fundamental redefinition periodically to stay current with changes in the larger operating environment (C).

The top stair in Figure 11.2 (upper right corner) represents the breakthrough vision and is labeled as the "Ideal Vision" of overall performance. The ideal vision may stretch as far as needed to illuminate the performance gap and thus establish creative tension. The bottom stair (lower left corner) is labeled "History/Mission." Understanding the history of the organization, department, service, or technology helps managers to identify and uncover issues, attitudes, or past events that may undermine implementation. An understanding of the past also promotes buy-in to change by grounding the change efforts through establishing continuity with past events (see Chapter 6). A clear statement of mission describes the purpose and justifies the existence of an organization, department, service, or process (see Chapter 8).

Connecting the bottom stair (History/Mission) with the top stair (Ideal Vision) are numerous steps that represent specific interventions or improvements designed to move performance closer to the ideal. The steps taken toward achieving the vision must not be so great as to prevent the care providers' focus and attention from being distracted and, in turn, placing patient safety and outcomes at risk (Reason 1990). However, the steps taken in implementation must be large enough so that slipping back to the previous way of doing things is not possible. Each step may have one intervention, or several concurrent interventions may exist per step. Some inter-

FIGURE 11.3
Incremental
Versus
Breakthrough
Improvements
in Technology

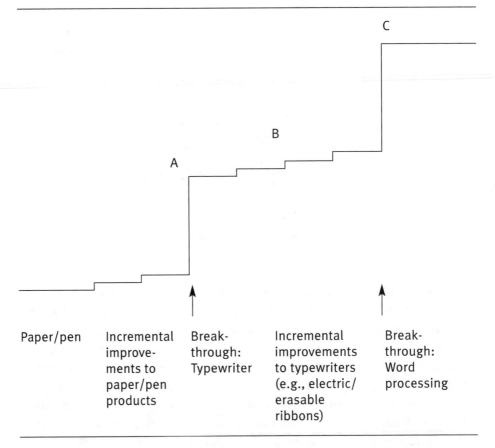

ventions may be completed quickly, and some may be broken down and achieved in several sequential steps, as shown in Figure 11.5. The diagonal line beneath the steps and pointing toward the ideal vision is labeled "Performance Measurement System," indicating that progress toward the vision is continually evaluated.

Figure 11.6 illustrates how the surgical services manager described in Chapter 7 implemented the unit's multiple goals in staged fashion according to this framework. The bottom step represents the mission of the service line. The top step on the right of the diagram represents the overall vision and the general goals. The performance measurement system is shown beneath the stairs and was the first intervention implemented. The first four steps represent specific interventions targeted toward restructuring the governance system to enhance collaboration, partnership, and decision making. Although not explicit in the performance goals, these interventions were essential to carrying out this manager's implicit goals to promote the desired culture needed for future interventions to succeed (see Chapter 7). Subsequent steps represent specific operational improvements that are based on how the multiple goals were defined (Kelly et al. 1997).

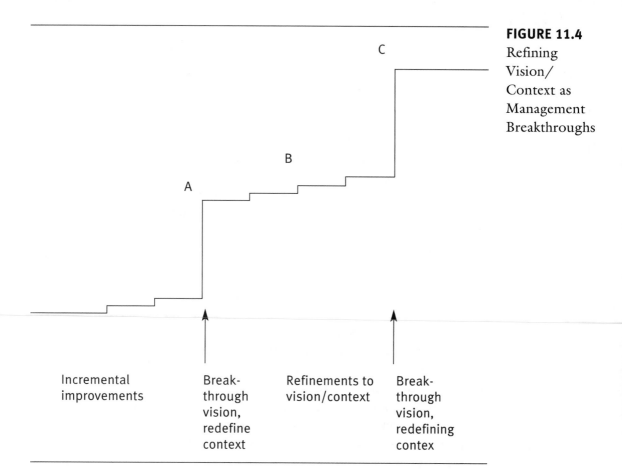

FIGURE 11.4
Refining
Vision/
Context as
Management
Breakthroughs

C

B

A

Incremental
improvements

Break-
through
vision,
redefine
context

Refinements to
vision/context

Break-
through
vision,
redefining
contex

The step below the top step is simply labeled "etc." The interventions shown in Figure 11.6 were only the beginning of the ongoing performance improvement culture. Short-term improvement goals, long-term improvement goals, and "just-do" interventions became an integral part of how this service line operated. The unit was also guided by performance gaps identified in the data and those gaps observed by staff and various governance team members (Kelly et al. 1997).

Figure 11.7 illustrates an example of how an improvement team from a medical-surgical unit in a small county hospital (see Chapter 7) documented its performance improvement efforts using the breakthrough vision, incremental implementation framework. Although not as large in scope as the previous example, this 30-bed patient care area found the framework helpful in organizing, documenting, and communicating its efforts. The first step in the lower left corner of the figure documents how the team reevaluated the unit's mission and scope of service and reviewed the unit's history at the beginning of the effort. The step in the upper right corner documents how the team defined its vision in terms of the characteristics

FIGURE 11.5
Breakthrough
Vision,
Incremental
Implementa-
tion: Staged
Implementa-
tion

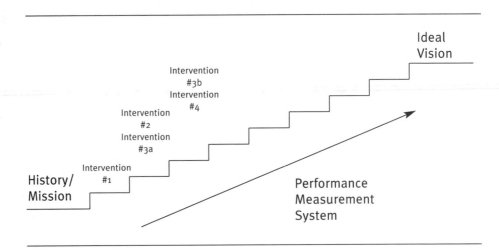

of its ideal unit. The team's performance measurement system is represented by the first diagonal arrow beneath the steps. This department already
had a set of clinical indicators in place but lacked financial, productivity,
and patient satisfaction measures. The first step represents the first intervention of devising a daily census and productivity report that enabled
charge nurses to more effectively allocate and assign staff resources.

When converted to a monthly report, this addition to the clinical
performance measures formed the basis of the team's performance measurement system. Recognizing that the patient satisfaction component of
its measurement plan would take a bit longer to operationalize, the team
worked on other interventions while refining and completing its performance measurement system.

Improvement interventions in this case focused on medium-term
goals of clarifying roles and worker expectations and integrating measurement into charge nurse decision making and staff meeting agendas. The
team also differentiated between short-term interventions—that is, its ongoing "Just-Do Action Plan" represented by the diagonal line beneath the
steps—and interventions that would take a bit longer to plan and implement, which are represented by the diagonal line labeled "Long-Term
Action Plan." Longer-term goals included addressing clinical processes of
care and other patient-related improvements. This team used the steps to
document the interventions already completed. They used the action plans
to track progress of ongoing interventions, and when an intervention was
completed, they added a new step to the diagram. The top step is labeled
"Future File"; the future file contained creative ideas that the team wanted
to remember but was not quite ready or able to pursue at the current time.

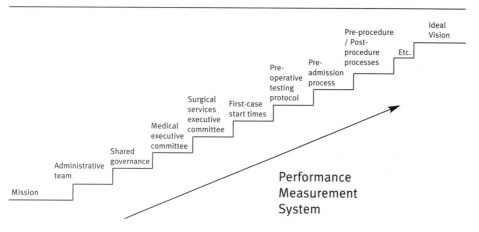

FIGURE 11.6
Breakthrough
Vision,
Incremental
Implementa-
tion: Surgical
Services

Source: Kelly, D. L., S. L. Pestotnik, M. C. Coons, and J. W. Lelis. 1997. "Reengineering a Surgical Service Line: Focusing on Core Process Improvement." *American Journal of Medical Quality* 12 (2): 120–29.

Conclusion

Implementing an improvement effort or a more comprehensive performance management system may at first appear intimidating to managers. However, by working backward from an ideal vision, the manager may begin to view the process in more manageable increments. Managers must also realize that implementation is not an isolated event when operating from a quality management philosophy but rather an ongoing way of conducting business.

The exercise at the end of this chapter provides the reader an opportunity to practice identifying mental models that may unintentionally undermine implementation efforts if communicated by management or through change and improvement processes. The exercise also provides a chance to practice identifying unintended consequences. Chapter 12 begins to explore practical team strategies that integrate an understanding of systems thinking.

Companion Readings

Dorner, D. 1996. *The Logic of Failure: Recognizing and Avoiding Error in Complex Situations,* 153–83. Reading, MA: Perseus Books.

Kelly, D., and D. Weber. 1995. "Creating an Environment for Participation in Healthcare." *Journal for Quality and Participation* 18 (7): 38–43.

FIGURE 11.7
Breakthrough
Vision,
Incremental
Implemen-
tation:
Medical-
Surgical Unit,
Rural County
Hospital

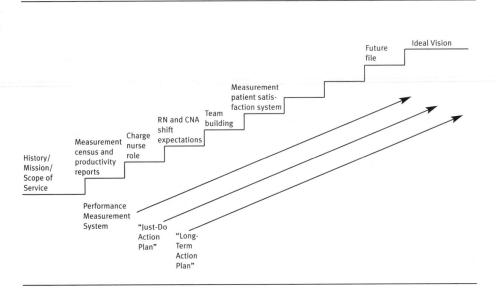

References

Covey, S. R. 1990. *The Seven Habits of Highly Effective People.* New York: Simon and Schuster.

Dorner, D. 1996. *The Logic of Failure: Recognizing and Avoiding Error in Complex Situations.* Reading, MA: Perseus Books.

James, B. C. 2001. "The Scientific Basis of Quality Improvement." Presentation to the 4th International Conference on the Scientific Basis of Healthcare, Sydney, Australia, September 22.

Kelly, D. L., S. L. Pestotnik, M. C. Coons, and J. W. Lelis. 1997. "Reengineering a Surgical Service Line: Focusing on Core Process Improvement." *American Journal of Medical Quality* 12 (2): 120–29.

Kofman, F., and P. Senge. 1993. "Communities of Commitment: The Heart of Learning Organizations." *Organizational Dynamics* 2 (2): 5–23.

Langley, G. J., K. M. Nolan, T. W. Nolan, C. L. Norman, and L. P. Provost. 1996. *The Improvement Guide: A Practical Approach to Enhancing Organizational Performance.* San Francisco: Jossey-Bass.

Nadler, G., and S. Hibino. 1994. *Breakthrough Thinking: The Seven Principles of Creative Problem Solving.* Rocklin, CA: Prima Publishing.

Reason, J. 1990. *Human Error.* Cambridge, MA: Cambridge University Press.

Exercise

Objectives:

- To practice identifying mental models reflected in selected management approaches
- To practice anticipating unintended consequences

Instructions:

1a. You are a manager faced with initiating an improvement effort. Two contrasting approaches to planning, launching the effort, selecting the team, and defining your role in the effort are shown below. Describe the assumptions or mental models conveyed by the different approaches. Write your responses on a worksheet similar to the one shown below.

Activity Model(s)	Approach Communicated	Assumption(s)/ Mental Model(s)	Approach Communicated	Assumption(s)/ Mental Model(s)
Planning	Planning by a guidance team composed of management		Integrate planning as part of the team process	
Launching the effort	Change announced by management		Provide information about the problem	
Selecting the team	Team members are appointed by the guidance team or selected by management		Management sets direction and boundaries for participation (e.g., how many, available funds); team members self-selected and/ or selected by their peers	
Defining the manager's/ facilitator's role	Directs the process; accountable for implementation and results		Manager is coach, trainer, information source, and barrier-buster; the entire team and/or system owns accountability for success	

1b. Select your preferred approach to each activity based on the messages that you would like your actions to communicate. You may select an original approach if desired. Describe your rationale for selecting that approach, and write your responses on a worksheet similar to the one below.

Activity	Preferred/Original Approach	Rationale
Planning		
Launching the effort		
Selecting the team		
Defining the manager's/ facilitator's role		

2. Record your responses for this exercise on a worksheet similar to the one below.
   a. Select any process that takes place within a healthcare organization. Write that process in the center column, Column A.
   b. Identify what/who influences the process in Column B.
   c. Identify what/who is influenced by the process in Column C.
   d. Extend your response one more time. Identify what/who influences the items in Column B. Write your response in Column D.
   e. Identify what/who is influenced by the items in Column C. Write your response in Column E.

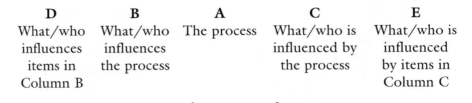

D	B	A	C	E
What/who influences items in Column B	What/who influences the process	The process	What/who is influenced by the process	What/who is influenced by items in Column C

   f. Describe one or two unintended consequences to a change in the process identified in Column A.

12

TEAM STRATEGIES

Objectives

- To explore practical team strategies
- To appreciate individuals' differences
- To practice identifying team member strengths

A s the department managers at Hospital A sat around the conference table, their minds were elsewhere. One was reviewing financial reports, one was reading mail, one was reviewing his weekly calendar, and one was in and out of the room answering phone calls. The administrator kept talking, oblivious to the indifference and apathy of the people in the room. Because attendance weighed heavily in the manager's performance appraisal, all managers attended the monthly management team meetings. According to anyone who was asked, the meetings were "a waste of time, but you have to go" to them.

The administrator at Hospital B started by reviewing the objective of the monthly management team meeting: to provide a forum for information sharing, learning, and collaborative problem solving and improvement. The team consisted of the managers within the administrator's scope of responsibility and the human resources, quality, and financial consultants dedicated to his service line. Each participant was leafing through the agenda packet as the administrator reviewed the items that will be discussed during the next two hours: "First, each manager will summarize his or her performance indicators for the month. The summary graphs for each department are in your packet, and so is the entire service line report. Please be sure to point out the positive trends and alert us to potential problems. Second on the agenda is a brief presentation from Manager A about the results of a recent improvement effort and what his team learned from the process. Finally, Manager B will summarize the important points from the conference he attended last week. Does anyone else have anything they need to add to the agenda?" At the conclusion of the meeting, the managers were still milling around the room, asking each other questions, laughing together, and competitively joking about whose performance statistics had shown the most improvement this year.

In both of these examples, highly paid managerial employees were brought together regularly for a meeting. However, the yield from each of these meetings differed. Predictably, the overall yield from each manager and from the service line as a whole also differed. The collective intelligence of the organization is often an under-recognized variable in the productivity equation, especially when applied to knowledge work like healthcare.

The ability to effectively design and manage teams is an essential management skill. The published literature already offers managers a wealth of information about teams, so this chapter will not review nor summarize them. This chapter, however, explores some practical team strategies related to the specific concepts described in this book.

Designing Teams

Effective teams do not just happen; they are thoughtfully and purposefully designed. Often the first question asked about a team is, "Who should be on it?" However, the following sequence of questions should be asked any time a manager is considering a team approach on any level, whether on a management team, a project team, a care delivery team, or an improvement team level.

1.   What is the purpose (e.g., of an activity, process, function)?
2.   What is the ideal, step-by-step process or approach to achieve that purpose?
3.   What is the most appropriate structure to support and carry out that process? (Structure includes how people are organized to carry out the process.)

Purpose

When the two meeting examples above are examined according to these three questions, we discover that the management team meetings in Hospital A did not have a purpose or a defined process. Although its structure was defined, without addressing the first two questions, this structure had little impact on manager effectiveness and, in turn, on departmental and organizational performance. In Hospital B, the purpose was clearly defined as providing a forum for information sharing, learning, and collaborative problem solving and improvement. The step-by-step process to achieve this purpose was a defined agenda at each meeting that included discussing performance indicators, sharing successes and individuals' learning, and communicating organizational information from administrator to managers, managers to administrator, and managers to managers. The team members included not only the managers but also a financial officer, a human resources consultant, and a quality department staff member assigned to the service line. They assisted with compiling the performance data, generating management reports, and answering data-related questions at the meetings. Guest speakers were invited to address special topics of discussion. The managers in this service line not only demonstrated a high level of individual performance and satisfaction, but the service line overall consistently demonstrated the highest level of relative improvement year after year.

In redesigning a clinical care team, the following questions should be asked:

- What is the purpose of care in this care setting?
- What is the process of care that will achieve this purpose?
- What is the structure (e.g., types and organization of care providers) needed to carry out this process?

Process

Aligning Messages

In one project team, the facilitator and manager would debrief after the team meeting to clarify their respective responsibilities for the next meeting. The agreed-on guidelines defined how the team would make decisions, but when the team members observed the manager and facilitator having a meeting after the meeting, they began to suspect that the manager had a hidden agenda and was influencing the facilitator toward his agenda rather than the team's agenda. When the unintended messages sent by the post-meeting meeting were realized, the manager clearly explained the assumptions behind his actions. The manager wanted to make sure that the team had the managerial support necessary to accomplish their goals. Depending on the meeting agenda and resulting discussion, the manager and facilitator often identified issues, information, or follow-up activities that the staff were unaware of because of the nature of their roles. For subsequent team efforts, the manager and facilitator adopted the practice of explaining very early in the project that they needed to discuss certain topics without the team. They hoped that this explanation would proactively prevent any misperceptions associated with "the meeting after the meeting."

Decision Making

Consensus is a widespread approach to decision making in which the team seeks to find a proposal acceptable enough that all members can support it (Scholtes, Joiner, and Streibel 1996). Seeking consensus may, however, reduce decisions to the lowest common denominator (Wheatley 1994). In a team comprising primarily concrete-, practical-, linear-thinking members, how likely is it that an idea posed by the one creative, conceptual team member would gain enough acceptance to be considered a possible solution to a problem? Or, conversely, on a team of creative, conceptual innovators quickly moving forward on an idea without regard for the practical considerations of implementation, how likely would the input from the one concrete-, practical-, linear-thinking team member be embraced? In either case, the result will be less than optimal. The best result (i.e., improvement intervention) in these two circumstances may come from listening to the "outlier" because that team member's perspective best matches the requirements of the decision at hand. Predictably, the first team showed minimal improvement after its idea was implemented, and the second team never was able to implement its idea.

Using decision criteria is an alternative to consensus. Using criteria does not imply that the team is not accountable for supporting a decision once it is made; it does, however, suggest that decisions will more likely take a diverse perspective into consideration. For example, in one improvement effort, the criteria for pursuing an improvement idea included the following (Kelly 1998):

- Does it fit within the goal of the effort?
- Does it meet customer requirements?
- Does it meet regulatory requirements?
- Does it remain consistent with the department's/organization's purpose?
- Does it support the vision?
- Does it demonstrate consistency with quality principles?

In this case, team members were expected to question and challenge an idea and, if an idea met the criteria, the team could pursue it further, confident that the idea was sound. Even though all team members did not completely understand the idea at the time, much time was saved in trying to explain something that was not readily understandable given the individual natures of the team members.

Meeting Schedules and Frequency

Typical meetings are held weekly, biweekly, or monthly, and they generally last one to two hours. Some of the challenges associated with this approach in healthcare organizations include clinical providers not being able to get away from daily patient care duties, team members arriving late because of other competing responsibilities, the need to devote portions of the meeting to update team members, and dwindling interest as the process drags on.

Consider an alternative approach. If managers use a systematic method for approaching improvements, they will begin to get a sense for the total team time required for an improvement effort. For example, a team may take about 40 hours to complete the various phases of an improvement project. If the improvement effort is constrained by time or dollars, the team is faced with increasing its own productivity or reducing its own cycle time. With this in mind, the 40 hours of time may be distributed in a variety of ways other than one- to two-hour segments. For example, ten four-hour meetings or five eight-hour meetings may better meet the needs of a particular project. The meetings may occur once a week for ten weeks, twice a week for five weeks, or every day for one week. Based on the particular work environment, a strategy may be selected that balances project team productivity, daily operational capacity and requirements, the scope of the desired improvement, and project deadlines.

A concentrated team meeting schedule has several advantages:

- it demonstrates the organization's or management's commitment to change,
- it saves duplication and rework associated with bringing everyone up to speed at each meeting,
- it establishes traction by contributing to the elements of creative tension,
- it reduces the cycle time from concept to implementation, and
- it forces managers and teams out of the "fire-fighting" mentality into one of purposely fixing not just symptoms of problems but the underlying problems themselves.

Structure

For an improvement project team, team composition (how many and who are on the team) as well as meeting frequency and duration should be guided by the purpose and team processes for the improvement effort. The questions that should be asked include, "What knowledge is required to design the actual improvement intervention(s)?" "How should the team be designed to support the processes needed to accomplish implementation within the project constraints?"

Focusing on early adopters has been shown to be an effective strategy to get individuals to adopt an innovation. Once approximately 5 to 20 percent of a group have successfully adopted a new process, adoption by the rest of the required group progresses very rapidly (Rogers 1995). According to the Myers-Briggs Type Indicator, approximately 68 percent of the population will express a personality type that is resistant to change, while 32 percent will express a type that is accepting of change (Myers, Kirby, and Myers 1998; Smith 2000). Within the two groups exists an entire continuum of resistance and acceptance. Typically, early adopters of innovations fall into specific Myers-Briggs types.

What does a manager do when faced with implementing improvements when very few early adopters are in the employee pool? This was the case for a manager who needed to obtain rapid buy-in for a large change effort in a department composed mostly of people with resistant personality types. The manager chose a strategy involving a 40-member improvement team, which represented about 25 percent of the total department staff; the team included formal and informal leaders in the department. Although most of these 40 people fell into the "resistant" group, by involving them earlier rather than later in the process, the manager not only engaged those who readily accepted change but also simultaneously cultivated the critical mass of the resistant types needed to support implementing the improvements. In this way, the speed with which the improvements were adopted and implemented throughout the entire department was greatly enhanced (Kelly 1998).

Team Effectiveness

Although agreement and harmony may be preferred by many managers and employees, the convergence of diverse perspectives is what supplies the essential elements of creative tension and potentially leads to innovation and improvement, as this quote indicates:

> Innovate or fall behind: the competitive imperative for virtually all businesses today is that simple. Achieving it is hard, however, because innovation takes place when different ideas, perceptions, and ways of processing and judging information collide. That, in turn, often requires collaboration among various players who see the world in inherently different ways. (Leonard and Straus 1997a)

Although diverse perspectives serve a role in creative tension and foster innovation, they also create fertile ground for accidental adversaries, conflict, and team breakdowns. Managers are challenged to find tools and approaches that enable them to take advantage of differing perspectives while maintaining effective interpersonal relationships within teams and employee groups. How can managers promote friction among ideas while minimizing friction among people?

Talents and Differences

Numerous frameworks are available to assist managers in understanding and appreciating individuals and their differences. Although the taxonomy may vary, each framework defines groups on the basis of common patterns. Studies of large numbers of individuals have resulted in the identification of patterns in their preferences, predispositions, temperaments, learning styles, and strengths. These patterns have been organized and labeled according to various frameworks, including the Myers-Briggs Type Indicator (Myers, Kirby, and Myers 1998), the Keirsey Temperament Sorter (Keirsey 1998), Human Dynamics (Seagal and Horne 1997), and the StrengthsFinder (Buckingham and Clifton 2001). Specific descriptions of these frameworks are not provided in this book, but readers are encouraged to further explore them; see the reference list at the end of the chapter.

When these different frameworks are studied together as a group, patterns may be identified. First, the frameworks recognize that individuals bring differences with them to the workplace. The frameworks identify, categorize, and explain those differences and then provide a concrete and systematic means of recognizing, describing, and understanding them. They also provide a common language and approach for managers and teams within the organization to understand, appreciate, and address differences in the workplace in a positive way. When two of these frameworks—the Myers-Briggs Type Indicator and Human Dynamics—are studied together, some global, cross-cutting dichotomies may also be seen. These include the following dualities: internal and external, practical and creative, data oriented and relationship oriented, concrete and conceptual, linear and lateral, and spontaneous and structured. Although managers may prefer one framework over another, they should begin to look for how these global dichotomies are expressed in themselves, in their employees, and within teams in their organization. Managing the interface of these dichotomies rather than avoiding or falling victim to them will enable managers to enhance the effectiveness of both operational working teams and improvement project teams.

Operational Teams

As patient volumes increased, a department grew from 5 employees to 20 almost overnight. With only five employees, the department functioned like a close-knit family. When new employees came on board, they found themselves thrown into the work with little time to assimilate into the culture and style of the team. For the first time, the department appointed a supervisor to oversee the team, and not long after that the complaints started—that is, the supervisor never follows through on anything, a certain employee is not carrying his or her load, the supervisor is all talk and no action.

This department had inadvertently set up an accidental adversaries situation between the supervisor and the staff. In Chapter 6, the term *accidental adversaries* was used in relation to double-loop learning and making underlying assumptions explicit. However, accidental adversaries as a result of differences in personalities, styles, and preferences can be a common and unrecognized source of conflict in all kinds of teams.

When the employees in this department took the Myers-Briggs Type Indicator test, the results were illuminating. Eighteen of the 20 department employees were *sensing* types. They preferred the concrete, real, factual, structured, and tangible here-and-now; they became impatient with the abstract and mistrusted intuition. Two of the employees, including the supervisor, were *intuitive* types. These two preferred possibilities, theories, invention, and the new; they enjoyed discussions characterized by spontaneous leaps of intuition, and they tended to leave out or neglect details (Myers, Kirby, and Myers 1998). In this department, the supervisor inherently functioned in a manner that was just about opposite to the rest of the department's inherent way of functioning. As a result, misunderstandings, misperceptions, and communication breakdowns became common.

When these differences were understood, the department could put into place specific processes and systems (which were not necessary with only a few employees) to minimize the potential breakdowns. For example, a standing agenda at staff meetings helped the supervisor to stay on task and avoid getting sidetracked. A bulletin board and communication notebook was used to ensure that current and complete information about departmental issues was available to everyone. A performance measurement system was put into place to provide a factual base for evaluating individual productivity and workload.

By understanding and implementing processes designed to meet the differing information and communication needs of the sensing and intuitive types, this department was able to avert further conflict and misunderstanding and focus employees' energy on productive work rather than on the perceived supervisory deficiencies.

Project Teams

Just as managers use human resources practices that promote matching an employee's traits with the requirements of the job, managers may also match employees with the various roles and stages required in a change or improvement process. Problems in group processes tend to arise from a mismatch between a process stage and an individual rather than from problems inherent in the individuals themselves. Purposefully engaging the individuals at the appropriate time in the process and offering support and requesting patience during other times can enhance the team's and the manager's effectiveness.

A team member favoring a concrete pattern may get frustrated with creating a vision, although he or she will be essential in determining the logistics of the implementation. Someone with an interpersonal or relational pattern can be on the alert for any employee issues related to the changes. An employee with a pattern of seeing the big picture will be invaluable in identifying unintended consequences. A team member who is detail oriented can be an ideal choice for monitoring progress and ensuring follow-through; another member who is action oriented can make sure the team gets moving.

Conclusion

When managers realize that individual mental models and organizational context surrounding the concepts described in this chapter influence how quality management is operationalized in an organization, they may gain a deeper appreciation for the value of teams as systemic structures. Managers should not only examine their individual mental models as a way to enhance their own personal effectiveness, but they should also incorporate an understanding of this systemic structure while defining the context of the work environment. The manager's responsibility is to select the desired lens through which individuals within the organization and the organization as a whole will view the world. A lens that views differences as complementary talents may result in synergy and success, while a lens that views differences as opposing perspectives may result in conflict, breakdowns, and mediocrity.

Often, team guidelines suggest rules of behavior such as "we will start on time" or "do not interrupt while another person is talking." The exercise at the end of this chapter offers an alternative approach to establishing team guidelines that enhance the team's ability to use team member strengths, increase the team's effectiveness, and improve the quality of the team's output.

Companion Readings

Rubin, I. 1996. "Learning How to Learn: The Key to CQI." *Physician Executive* 22 (10): 22–27.

Seagal, S., and D. Horne. 1994. "Human Dynamics: A Foundation for the Learning Organization." *The Systems Thinker* 5 (4): 1–4.

References

Buckingham, M., and D. O. Clifton. 2001. *Now, Discover Your Strengths.* New York: The Free Press.

Keirsey, D. 1998. *Please Understand Me II: Temperament Character Intelligence.* Del Mar, CA: Prometheus Nemesis Book Company.

Kelly, D. L. 1998. "Reframing Beliefs About Work and Change Processes in Redesigning Laboratory Services." *Joint Commission Journal on Quality Improvement* 24 (9): 154–67.

Leonard, D., and S. Straus. 1997. "Putting Your Company's Whole Brain to Work." *Harvard Business Review* 75 (4): 110–19.

Myers, I. B., L. K. Kirby, and K. D. Myers. 1998. *Introduction to Type: A Guide to Understanding Your Results on the Myers-Briggs Type Indicator.* Palo Alto, CA: Consulting Psychologists Press, Inc.

Rogers, E. M. 1995. *Diffusion of Innovations.* New York: The Free Press.

Scholtes, P. R., B. L. Joiner, and B. J. Streibel. 1996. *The Team Handbook,* 2nd Edition. Madison, WI: Joiner Associates, Inc.

Seagal, S., and D. Horne. 1997. *Human Dynamics: A New Framework for Understanding People and Realizing the Potential in Our Organizations.* Cambridge, MA: Pegasus Communications, Inc.

Smith, R. 2000. *The Seven Levels of Change: The Guide to Innovation in the World's Largest Corporations.* Arlington, TX: The Summit Publishing Group.

Wheatley, M. J. 1994. *Self-Organizing Systems: The New Science of Change.* Kelner-Rogers and Wheatley, Inc. Conference Proceedings, Deer Valley, Utah, October 17–19.

Exercise

Objective: To practice establishing team guidelines that capitalize on the strengths of team members

Note: Part I of this exercise may be used to start any group or team discussion. Parts II and III are designed to be used midway through and at the end of a defined team process or project.

Instructions:

1. Assign roles in your group. These roles may stay the same or rotate among team members to provide an opportunity for each team member to practice each role.
    *   Select a leader. The leader is responsible for ensuring that the group expectations are completed within the time allotted and that too much time is not spent on one item.
    *   Select a scribe. The scribe is responsible for recording the highlights of the discussion.
    *   Select a timekeeper. The timekeeper will keep the group informed about how much time remains for the meeting or session.
2. Select and agree on group rules. These rules represent guidelines and expectations for how individuals and the group will function to promote the accomplishment of the team's assignment. As a start, the following rules are suggested:
    *   Give your full attention.
    *   Be respectful of others.
    *   Accept responsibility for the team's success.

    Add additional group rules as desired.
    *
    *
    *
3. Identify and discuss each team member's strengths and limitations. Record these characteristics on the following worksheet. Use this worksheet as a reference for your team.

Part I: Team Member Strengths Worksheet

Name	My unique contribution to this project team (e.g., experience, education, perspective, skill, background)	What I am least effective at doing (it is not that I am unwilling to try, it is just not my strength)

Part II: Midway Team Evaluation and Improvement Plan Worksheet

Scoring Guidelines: 3 = Very effective, 2 = Somewhat effective, 1 = Needs improvement

Item	Score		Improvement Plan
	Individual	Group	
Following team guidelines			
• Giving your full attention			
• Being respectful of others			
• Accepting responsibility for the team's success			
•			
•			
The degree to which team member strengths were contributed:			
Name:			
Name:			
Name:			
Name:			
Name:			
The degree to which team member limitations were minimized:			
Name:			
Name:			
Name:			
Name:			
Name:			

Part III: Final Team Evaluation Worksheet

Instructions: Review your midway team evaluation and improvement plan. Complete the final team evaluation.

Scoring Guidelines: 3 = Very effective, 2 = Somewhat effective, 1 = Needs improvement

Item	Midway Evaluation Score		Final Evaluation Score	
	Individual	Group	Individual	Group
Following team guidelines				
• Giving your full attention				
• Being respectful of others				
• Accepting responsibility for the team's success				
•				
•				
The degree to which team member strengths were contributed:				
Name:				
Name:				
Name:				
Name:				
Name:				
The degree to which team member limitations were minimized:				
Name:				
Name:				
Name:				
Name:				
Name:				

EPILOG

The concepts and tools examined in this book come from varied disciplines, yet each has its origins in systems perspective. When used together, their synergy provides managers with a guide to leveraging performance improvement and change efforts. The concept of leverage is derived from physics and is defined as "an advantage for accomplishing a purpose" or an "increased power of action" (Oxford English Dictionary 2003). Leverage is achieved through the action of a lever, which is defined as "a bar used for prying" or "an inducing or compelling force" (Merriam-Webster Online 2003).

In the past, quality management in healthcare has focused on tools to enhance a manager's ability to improve how processes are carried out (process) and to improve the work that is carried out (content). In the future, managers will be required also to employ tools that examine underlying thinking and assumptions. This book has provided managers with a set of tools that can prepare them for future demands for improvement within healthcare. The tools are intended to address high-leverage, underlying assumptions (i.e., systemic structures) that influence quality management. These assumptions relate to goals, purpose, measurement, traction, implementation, and teams. The figure on the next page illustrates the continuum from low- to high-leverage performance improvement.

A manager must know when to accept and when to challenge underlying assumptions to succeed in an uncertain environment. The ability to understand and fluidly manage the relationship between traditional quality tools and tools that provide a deeper understanding of assumptions and other underlying systemic structures permits the manager to continually raise the quality management lever bar.

When asked how to get to Carnegie Hall, a famous musician replied, "practice, practice, practice!" The exercises at the end of each chapter provide the reader an opportunity to practice the presented concepts and tools. The exercises in the next section offer the reader an opportunity to further synthesize these concepts and tools by applying them to a performance improvement effort in a healthcare organization setting.

FIGURE
Leveraging
Performance
Improvement
in Healthcare

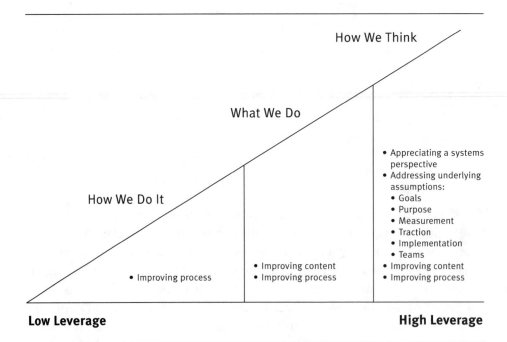

References

Merriam-Webster Online. 2003. [Online information; retrieved 2/25/03]. www.m-w.org.

Oxford English Dictionary. 2003. [Online information; retrieved 2/25/03]. http://dictionary.oed.com.

PRACTICE EXERCISES

Practice is crucial in any improvement effort. The exercises in this section allow readers to refine their understanding of and familarity with the theories and processes addressed in the book. The first exercise focuses readers on conducting an organizational assessment to document their organization's current reality. The second exercise involves students in a performance improvement effort in a fictional organization with real-world organizational conflicts. The third exercise allows managers to practice a performance improvement on identified areas of their own organizations using the concepts and tools in this book.

Exercise 1

Objectives:

- To practice using an organizational assessment as a means of documenting current reality
- To practice using the Baldrige National Quality Program Healthcare Criteria for Performance Excellence as a guide for completing an organizational assessment

Notes:
1. Students may complete this exercise using the "CapStar Health System Case Study" (see http://www.baldrige.gov/ASQ_Materials.htm). Working managers may complete this exercise using their own organizations as examples.
2. This exercise is adapted from the Baldrige National Quality Program Examiner Workbook (see http://www.baldrige.gov/02scorebook.htm) and the Baldrige National Quality Program Health Care Criteria for Performance Excellence (see http://www.baldrige.gov/HealthCare_Criteria.htm).

3. For additional reference, please see D. L. Kelly. 2002. "Using the Baldrige Criteria for Improving Performance in Public Health." Doctoral dissertation. © UMI Company UMI Dissertation Services, Proquest, Ann Arbor, Michigan.

Instructions:

1. Select and describe boundaries of the system of interest; the term "organization" will be used to refer to this selected system. You may select a team, a department, a small organization (e.g., an office practice), or an entire organization.

2. Address the following categories within the organization: organizational profile, leadership, strategic planning, patient focus, information and analysis, staff focus, process management, and organizational performance results. Each of these areas is defined in the Organizational Assessment Worksheet.

3. Read the description of each of category (see worksheet). These descriptions represent the excellence indicators in the BNQP Healthcare Criteria for Performance. Identify one to three things that your organization does well, according to the excellence indicators. Write those strengths on a worksheet similar to the one provided.

4. Identify one to three things that you think your organization can do better, according to the excellence indicators. Write those opportunities for improvement on a worksheet similar to the one provided.

5. Refer to the BNQP Healthcare Criteria for Performance Excellence if you need a more detailed description of organizational activities that represent excellence indicators.

6. Select a priority area for improvement. You may use the Prioritizing Improvement Opportunities Worksheet provided, or you may write your responses on a worksheet similar to it.

Organizational Assessment Worksheet

Organizational Profile

This category is a snapshot of your organization, the key influences that affect how it operates, and the key challenges that it faces.

- Briefly describe your organization, including its services; its size; its geographic community; its key patient or customer groups; the number of patients it serves; and its current facilities, equipment, and technology.

- Briefly describe your organization's key challenges.

Leadership

This category examines how your organizational leaders address values, directions, and performance expectations as well as how focused they are on customers, stakeholders, empowerment, innovation, and learning. This category also examines how your organization addresses its responsibilities to the public and how it supports the community.

- Based on the above indicators, describe one to three key strengths of your organization's leadership.

- Based on the above indicators, describe one to three areas in which your organization's leadership can improve.

Strategic Planning

This category examines how your organization develops strategic objectives and action plans and how progress toward your chosen strategic objectives is measured.

- Based on the above indicators, describe one to three key strengths of your organization's strategic planning.

- Based on the above indicators, describe one to three areas of your organization's strategic planning that can be improved.

Focus on Patients, Other Customers, and Markets

This category examines how your organization determines requirements, expectations, and preferences of patients, other customers, and markets. It also examines how your organization builds relationships with patients and other customers and determines the key factors that lead to their acquisition, satisfaction, loyalty, and retention and to healthcare service expansion.

- Based on the above indicators, describe one to three key strengths in how your organization focuses on patients, other customers, and markets.

- Based on the above indicators, describe one to three opportunities that your organization can take to improve how it focuses on patients, customers, and markets.

Measurement, Analysis, and Knowledge Management

This category examines how your organization selects, gathers, analyzes, manages, and improves its data, information, and knowledge assets.

- Based on the above indicators, describe one to three key strengths of your organization's measurement, analysis, and knowledge management approaches.

- Based on the above indicators, describe one to three opportunities that your organization can take to improve its measurement, analysis, and knowledge management approaches.

Staff Focus

This category examines how your organization's work systems and staff learning and motivation enable all staff to develop and utilize their full potential in alignment with your organization's overall objectives and action plans. It also examines the organization's efforts to build and maintain a work environment and a staff support climate conducive to performance excellence and to personal and organizational growth.

- Based on the above indicators, describe one to three key strengths in how your organization demonstrates staff focus.

- Based on the above indicators, describe one to three opportunities that your organization can take to improve its staff focus.

Process Management

This category examines the key aspects of your organization's process management, including key healthcare, business, and other support processes for creating value for patients, other customers, and the organization. This category encompasses all key processes and all departments and work units.

- Based on the above indicators, describe one to three key strengths of your organization's process management.

- Based on the above indicators, describe one to three opportunities that your organization can take to improve its process management.

Organizational Performance Results

This category examines your organization's performance and improvement in key areas: healthcare delivery and outcomes, patient and other customer satisfaction, healthcare services, financial and marketplace performance, staff and work system results, operational performance, and governance and social responsibility. This area also examines performance levels relative to those of competitors and other organizations providing similar healthcare services.

- Describe one to three key areas in which your organization demonstrates strong performance, and describe the nature of the data that document these performance areas.

- Describe one to three areas in which your organization can improve performance and why you selected these performance areas.

Prioritizing Improvement Opportunities Worksheet

1. Review your opportunities for improvement in each organizational area described in the previous worksheet.
2. Select as a priority one of the opportunities for improvement in the area of Organizational Performance Results.
3. Explain below why you made this selection.
4. List any other opportunities for improvement (#1) that influence or are influenced by your selected priority for improvement (#2).
   -
   -
   -

Exercise 2

Objectives:

- To provide an opportunity for students to synthesize the concepts by being involved in a performance improvement effort using a case study that presents real conflicts in organizations.
- To practice in a safe and controlled setting

Notes:
1. This exercise is designed for five teams of students. Teams may elect to tackle one of the five performance gaps presented in the case study.
2. The following case study is not a business case study, which is a detailed description and account of the organization. Rather, it presents enough organizational context in which the concepts and tools described in this book can be applied.

Instructions:

1. Read the case study and answer the questions afterward. The questions do not require you to have all the answers, but they lead you to ask the right questions. If you think you need more content information on certain areas (i.e., details about the organization or data), identify that need by defining the questions you would ask to obtain that information.

Case Study

Background

You work in a large community hospital. Last year, the hospital admitted 20,925 inpatients. For 1,000 of these total patient admissions, congestive heart failure (CHF) was documented as the primary or secondary diagnosis. Of these CHF patients, 48 percent are female and 52 percent are male. The mean age of the CHF patients is 63 years old. Approximately 50 percent have a history of CHF, while approximately 50 percent are newly diagnosed. The average length of stay for a CHF patient with a primary or secondary diagnosis is 5.6 days. The payer mix for the group is 50 percent Medicare, 40 percent private, and 10 percent indigent or charity. As part of the hospital's three- to five-year plan to excel in cardiac services, the hospital will focus on CHF as one of its goals this year.

Clinical Performance Gap

Your team represents internists and other clinical staff in an internal medicine practice. Your combined interest in improving outcomes in patients with CHF prompted you to join an improvement project sponsored by your state quality improvement organization. As part of the project, you helped to clarify guidelines for this patient population in the areas of diagnosis, treatment, and self-management education. Each of the team members has been using these guidelines for the past year.

You have received the evaluation data for the project that show the performance in the heart failure indicators required by the Centers for Medicare and Medicaid Services. The report shows your hospital's overall performance. You also receive individual reports showing how your patients compare. Your performance is 10 to 20 percent better in each of the indicators as compared with that of the hospital as a whole.

At the request of the hospital's medical staff president, you give a report on your project at the next medical staff meeting. Of the 1,000 CHF admissions a year, your patients represent only one-tenth of these admissions but demonstrate the best outcomes. At the end of the report, the medical staff president asks your team to lead an effort to improve care to all patients admitted to the hospital with a primary or secondary diagnosis of CHF.

Operational Performance Gap

Your team collectively represents the manager of the social work department at the hospital. At the monthly staff meeting, you ask your staff for input on the increasing overtime hours that you have observed on the payroll reports. The staff describe their frustrations with how discharge planning is being done at the hospital. With the trend toward shorter hospital stays, they are finding that they have more to do in less time. Responsibilities such as arranging transportation, ensuring follow-up appointments, and arranging home and long-term care are becoming more difficult.

Patients who come in for CHF and spend a day or two in the intensive care unit pose a particular problem. Many times, the social workers are not notified until the day the patient is supposed to be going home. As a result, everything becomes an emergency, which makes it hard for the social workers to manage their time effectively. You tell your staff that you will initiate an improvement effort on the discharge process and that you will begin with patients with CHF.

Operational Performance Gap

Your team collectively represents the nursing shift supervisors of the hospital. A nursing supervisor is assigned to each shift and has the responsibility for clinical and administrative oversight of the nursing staff for that shift. Your specific responsibilities include monitoring and ensuring adequate nursing staff coverage on each shift; serving as a resource to unit charge nurses; assisting with emergencies, such as codes; serving as the administrative liaison for patient complaints that are out of the ordinary or that unit staff are unable to handle; ensuring that admissions, transfers, and discharges of patients between units or departments occur smoothly; and helping to resolve interdepartmental conflicts.

Recently, in an effort to cut costs, the hospital approved a proposal to eliminate the day-shift supervisor. The rationale was that the patient care unit managers (a combination of traditional head nurses and the newer, nonclinical administrative managers) are present during the day and should be able to jointly absorb the functions of the shift supervisor. Since this change was implemented, your jobs on the evening and night shift have become more difficult. Patients who should have been discharged in the morning are being delayed until the afternoon. Because your bed capacity is typically around 80 percent, these delays are causing bottlenecks for new admissions from surgery and from the emergency department. The general medicine floors in particular—including the telemetry unit where the CHF patients are and where approximately 70 percent of the admissions come through the emergency department—are faced with these problems. You have heard the following comments from nurses throughout the hospital:

- "The managers seem to always be at meetings and are never available, so it's like not having a supervisor on day shift."
- "When I take the patients downstairs to the lobby to go home, I have always stopped at the outpatient pharmacy to get their prescriptions filled. Lately I have had to wait in line for 45 minutes!"
- "The doctors won't discharge patients until they see the morning blood work results. Since the lab work isn't drawn until 8:00 a.m., by the time I get the results back and track down the doctor to get the OK for discharge, it's usually close to noon."

Administrative Performance Gap

Your team collectively represents the administrator for the cardiac service line. The following departments report to you: the medicine/telemetry unit, the coronary care unit, the thoracic intensive care unit (i.e., heart surgery), the cardiac rehabilitation unit, the cardiac catheterization laboratory, and the EKG and echo laboratories. You are also the administrative liaison to the cardiologists and thoracic surgeons.

Because the nursing department is decentralized, you have a nursing director dedicated to your service line. She has just left your office after describing the complaints she has been receiving from the emergency department: patients are backing up in the emergency department as a result of delays in admitting patients to the general medicine floors, particularly the telemetry unit. The emergency department reports to the administrator responsible for the trauma service line.

You have just been recruited from out of state and are new to this position. You were hired with the expectation that you would improve the coordination of care for patients in your service line. The managers that report to you get together monthly for a managers' meeting. So far you have learned that these meetings have not been very useful in assisting managers with the issues that they consider important. Your predecessor had a traditional command-and-control style, and the managers feel stifled when making the improvements that they want to in their respective departments. You want to help your managers be more effective both individually and as a team.

Leadership Performance Gap

Your team represents the CEO of the hospital. You have been in the position for the last ten years, and your previous position was as a senior administrator. In the last few years, your job has become much more difficult: patients are sicker, lengths of stay are shorter, compliance and other regulations keep accumulating, staff turnover is increasing, and workforce shortages are more prevalent. Every time you go to a professional meeting, you hear of another colleague who has been "reorganized" out of a job. You feel fortunate to have remained in your position for so long, but at the last board meeting, the board made it clear that the hospital's performance must pick up. Your responsibility is to ensure that the board's requests are carried out. At first this expectation seems unreasonable, given that so many things are not under your control, like the nursing shortage. You remember going through a similar crisis in the 1990s, and you thought you had fixed it back then.

Since returning from an executive leadership conference a few weeks ago, you have been doing a lot of soul searching. Your management approach has always worked in the past, but it does not seem to be working anymore. You were intrigued by one of the keynote speakers at the conference, who described the attributes required by healthcare leaders today. A good leader is one whom others trust and have confidence in following because of that leader's values, vision, capabilities, and expertise in handling unstable and difficult situations; management of frustration, anxiety, and conflict are particularly admired. Such a leader keeps human suffering as the uppermost concern and enables groups to effectively manage surprises. A truly good leader is able to identify and help guide innovative projects through various forums such as strategic, scientific, economic/business, and political. The leader required in healthcare today has detailed knowledge of a variety of disciplines required to make a healthcare organization work well and has an insatiable curiosity to learn those disciplines that are unfamiliar (Peirce 2000).

You decide that starting today you will reinvent yourself in an effort to meet the board's expectations.

Questions

1. Select the performance gap that you will improve. Define, in a few sentences, the performance gap and the process(es) that contribute to this performance area.
2. Describe the customers and their expectations of this process or how you would get them (Voice of the Customer).
3. Select one of the systems models (see Chapter 5). Explain how the process(es) described in #1 fit(s) within the system illustrated by this model.
4. State the goal of the improvement effort. You may use the goals worksheet in Chapter 7 if it will help you organize your thinking.
5. Practice the purpose principle by asking yourself the following questions:
   - What am I trying to accomplish?
   - Have I expanded the purposes of addressing the problem? The purpose of (my previous response) is to . . . ?
   - Have I further expanded the purpose? The purpose of (my previous response) is to . . . ?
   - Have I further expanded the purpose? The purpose of (my previous response) is to . . . ?
   - Have I further expanded the purpose? The purpose of (my previous response) is to . . . ? (Continue expanding the purpose, if needed.)
   - What larger purpose may eliminate the need to achieve this smaller purpose altogether?
   - What is the right purpose for me to be working on? (Describe how this purpose differs or does not differ from the original purpose.)
6. Review the goal from #4. After completing the purpose questions in #5, does this still seem to be an appropriate goal? If not, redefine the goal of your improvement effort.
7. Describe a performance measure for this process (Voice of the Process) and how the data are collected. Create a control chart of this performance measure.
8. Describe the high-level steps of your process using a flowchart.
9. Practice identifying mental models.
   - Identify at least two mental models that may be interfering with achieving a higher level of performance from your process.
   - Describe an alternative mental model for each that may enhance the improvement of your process.
10. Describe your ideal vision for this process. Depending on the focus of your improvement, you may do this for the organization or department as a whole and then for an ideal process that is aligned with the overall vision. To assist in creating your vision, you may ask yourself the following questions:

If your process was the best practice for the community,
- What would your process contribute to the overall organizational performance and effectiveness?
- What would patients and families who are receiving care as a result of/influenced by your process say about their experience with your organization?
- What would employees involved in your process say about the process?
- What would colleagues around the country who came to learn from your best practice say about your process?

11. Improve your process.
- Determine if you are solving a problem associated with an existing process or creating a new process.
- Review your original and/or revised improvement goal(s).
- Review the purpose of your process.
- Review your customers' expectations.
- Review the mental models you selected.
- Identify any continuous quality improvement tools (see Chapter 3) that may assist you in better understanding how to improve your process.
- Define the starting and ending points of your process. Redefine them as needed to support the purpose.
- Based on the above information, describe your ideal process that will achieve the purpose you described. Document your process using a high-level flowchart.
- Check your process against the goal you set for your improvement effort.

12. Review the measure from #7 that you selected as the Voice of the Process. Is this measure still appropriate for your ideal process? If not, what would that measure be?

13. Review your goal and your purpose. Would the above measure(s) help you determine if you are working toward your goal and carrying out your purpose?

14. Describe any unintended consequences to any other area, department, process, or entity within or outside of your organization if you improve performance of your process. What measure(s) would help you to be on the alert for them?

15. Describe how the measure(s) from #12 and #13 fit into a balanced set of performance measures for the department or organization.

16. For your defined measures, describe the following:
- If the measure(s) is/are a process, outcome, or structure measure(s)
- Where the data for the measure(s) can be found or who to contact in the organization to find them
- How you would collect the data

- How often you would report the data
- What your control charts would look like
- With whom and how would you share your control charts

17. You have defined the purpose and described the ideal process. Determine the ideal structure to carry out this process—that is, who and how should the process be carried out to best achieve the purpose?

18. Describe an implementation plan that takes into consideration the concepts described in Chapter 11.

Reference

Peirce, J. C. 2000. "The Paradox of Physicians and Administrators in Healthcare Organizations." *Healthcare Management Review* 25 (1): 7–28.

Exercise 3

Objectives:

- To provide an opportunity for managers to synthesize the concepts by being involved in a performance improvement effort using the actual identified needs in their own organizations
- To practice in a safe and controlled setting

Note: Implementing the results of this exercise in your own organization is not required. However, the exercise requires that you think through and document all of the steps in the exercise as if you were actually conducting this effort in your organization.

Instructions:

1. Choose a performance gap or area for improvement based on the organizational assessment in Exercise 1. This should be an area for which you have access to performance data. (If actual performance data are not currently available, you need to define a plan of how to obtain it.) This should be an area that is key to your business strategy and within the scope of your defined business unit or responsibilities.
2. Briefly define the performance gap and the process(es) that contribute to this performance area.
3. Describe the customers and their expectations of this process or how you would get them (Voice of the Customer).
4. Select one of the systems models (see Chapter 5). Explain how the process(es) described in #2 fit(s) within the system illustrated by this model.
5. State the goal of the improvement effort. You may use the goals worksheet from Chapter 7 if it will help you to organize your thinking.
6. Practice the purpose principle by asking yourself the following questions:
   - What am I trying to accomplish?
   - Have I expanded the purposes of addressing the problem? The purpose of (my previous response) is to . . . ?
   - Have I further expanded the purpose? The purpose of (my previous response) is to . . . ?
   - Have I further expanded the purpose? The purpose of (my previous response) is to . . . ?
   - Have I further expanded the purpose? The purpose of (my previous response) is to . . . ? (Continue expanding the purpose, if needed.)
   - What larger purpose may eliminate the need to achieve this smaller purpose altogether?

- What is the right purpose for me to be working on? (Describe how this purpose differs or does not differ from the original purpose.)

7. Review the goal from #5. After completing the purpose questions in #6, does this still seem to be an appropriate goal? If not, redefine the goal of your improvement effort.

8. Describe a performance measure for this process (Voice of the Process) and how the data are collected. Create a control chart of this performance measure.

9. Describe the high-level steps of your process using a flowchart.

10. Practice identifying mental models.
    - Identify at least two mental models that may be interfering with achieving a higher level of performance from your process.
    - Describe an alternative mental model for each that may enhance the improvement of your process.

11. Practice infusing a different way of thinking into your improvement process.
    - Identify someone in your organization who appears to think in a different way than you do. Using the descriptions in Chapter 12, explain what led you to choose this person.
    - Review with this person your progress so far on this exercise
    - Ask this person for his or her perspective and critique. Describe how this perspective complemented or contradicted your own.
    - Describe how you will or will not incorporate this new perspective into your improvement process.

12. Describe your ideal vision for this process. Depending on the focus of your improvement, you may do this for the organization or department as a whole and then for an ideal process that is aligned with the overall vision. To assist in creating your vision, you may ask yourself the following questions:

    If your process was the best practice for the community,
    - What would your process contribute to the overall organizational performance/effectiveness?
    - What would patients and families who are receiving care as a result of/influenced by your process say about their experience with your organization?
    - What would employees involved in your process say about the process?
    - What would colleagues around the country who came to learn from your best practice say about your process?

13. Improve your process.
    - Determine if you are solving a problem associated with an exist-

ing process or creating a new process.

- Review your original and/or revised improvement goal(s).
- Review the purpose of your process.
- Review your customers' expectations.
- Review the mental models you selected.
- Identify any continuous quality improvement tools (see Chapter 3) that may assist you in better understanding how to improve your process.
- Define the starting and ending points of your process. Redefine them as needed to support the purpose.
- On the basis of the above information, describe your ideal process that will achieve the purpose you described. Document your process using a high-level flowchart.
- Check your process against the goal you set for your improvement effort.

14. Review the measure from #8 that you selected as the Voice of the Process. Is this measure still appropriate for your ideal process? If not, what would that measure be?

15. Review your goal and your purpose. Will the above measure(s) help you determine if you are working toward your goal and carrying out your purpose?

16. Describe any unintended consequences to any other area, department, process, or entity within or outside of your organization if you improve performance of your process. What measure(s) would help you to be on the alert for them?

17. Describe how the measure(s) from #14 and #15 fit into a balanced set of performance measures for the department/organization.

18. For your defined measures, describe the following:
    - If the measure(s) is/are a process, outcome, or structure measure(s)
    - Where the data for the measure(s) can be found or who to contact in the organization to find them
    - How you would collect the data
    - How often you would report the data
    - What your control charts would look like
    - With whom and how you would share your control charts

19. You have defined the purpose and described the ideal process. Determine the ideal structure to carry out this process—that is, who and how should the process be carried out to best achieve the purpose?

20. Describe an implementation plan that takes into consideration the concepts described in Chapter 11.

JOURNAL EXERCISE

Although reflection plays an important role in personal learning, it is not practiced often in today's demanding work environments. This journal exercise section provides the reader a structured opportunity for reflection on how the concepts discussed and the readings recommended in this book can be applied to circumstances and challenges in the actual work setting.

The questions posed in the journal-entry sheet serve three purposes. First, asking the reader to identify key points to remember allows him or her to personalize his or her own learning. Depending on the reader's experience and current circumstances, one topic may be particularly relevant to one reader, while the same concept may be repetitive or routine to another reader. This question asks the reader what lessons are important to him or her rather than instructs the reader to consider someone else's perspective.

Second, asking the reader to list the questions that arise as a result of the readings emphasizes the importance of posing questions. As managers and leaders mature in their roles, they discover that asking the right questions is essential to their effectiveness. Although readers, particularly students, may be accustomed to striving for the correct answers, they should know that this journal question is intended to encourage the practice of formulating good questions.

Finally, asking the reader how the concepts offered can be applied to his or her career roles, goals, and effectiveness helps solidify the main focus of this book: to apply quality management.

JOURNAL ENTRY

Name:_____ Date:_____

Title:

Author:

Source:

Number of pages:

1. Key points that I would like to remember from this reading. *(Write at least one point, but no more than five.)*:

    a.

    b.

    c.

    d.

    e.

2. New questions that I have as a result of this reading. *(Write at least one question, but no more than three.)*:

    a.

    b.

    c.

3. I can use the information from this reading in the following way. *(Be specific, and write no more than three to five sentences. Your answers may be related to your work role, your career goals, or your personal effectiveness.)*:

INDEX

ABOUT THE AUTHOR

Diane L. Kelly, Dr.P.H., M.B.A, R.N., is adjunct assistant professor at the University of North Carolina at Chapel Hill School of Public Health, where she teaches master's students in health policy and administration and public health leadership. She also serves as faculty for continuing professional educational programs, including Project HOPE's Health Care Management training program in Eastern Europe.

Dr. Kelly holds a BSN from West Virginia University, an MBA from University of Utah, and a Dr.P.H. in public health leadership from the University of North Carolina. Dr. Kelly's education and extensive clinical experience, including 20 years at Intermountain Health Care, allow her to offer a hands-on, patient- and practitioner-friendly teaching and facilitation style.

Dr. Kelly served as a member of the board of examiners for the Baldrige National Quality Program from 1999 to 2001. Her efforts have been the subject of peer-reviewed articles and other publications nationwide, including in the *Wall Street Journal*. As president of Emergent Solutions in Health Care, Dr. Kelly uses action-learning strategies to increase leadership capabilities in healthcare organizations.